# Our Country Nurse

Can East End Nurse Sarah
make a new life caring for
babies in the country?

# SARAH BEESON MBE
## WITH AMY BEESON

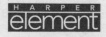

HARPER
element

HarperElement
An imprint of HarperCollins*Publishers*
1 London Bridge Street
London SE1 9GF

www.harpercollins.co.uk

First published by HarperElement 2016

1 3 5 7 9 10 8 6 4 2

© Sarah Beeson MBE and Amy Beeson 2016

Sarah Beeson MBE and Amy Beeson assert the moral
right to be identified as the authors of this work

A catalogue record of this book is
available from the British Library

ISBN 978-0-00-752009-1

Printed and bound in Great Britain by
Clays Ltd, St Ives plc

All rights reserved. No part of this publication may be
reproduced, stored in a retrieval system, or transmitted,
in any form or by any means, electronic, mechanical,
photocopying, recording or otherwise, without the
prior permission of the publishers.

FSC™ is a non-profit international organisation established to promote
the responsible management of the world's forests. Products carrying the
FSC label are independently certified to assure consumers that they come
from forests that are managed to meet the social, economic and
ecological needs of present and future generations,
and other controlled sources.

Find out more about HarperCollins and the environment at
www.harpercollins.co.uk/green

*In memory of the late*
*May Paulus, Desiree Knox Whyte and Pat Wrennall:*
*wonderful health visitors, mentors and friends*

# About Sarah Beeson

In 1969 17-year-old Sarah Beeson – then Sarah Hill – arrived in Hackney in the East End of London to begin her nursing career. Six years later she went into health visiting, practising for over 35 years in Kent and Staffordshire, building up a lifetime's expertise and stories through working with babies and families.

In 1998 Sarah received the Queen's Institute for Nursing Award. In 2006 she was awarded an MBE for Services to Children and Families by Queen Elizabeth II.

She later married and became Sarah Beeson. Now she divides her time between Staffordshire and London.

# About Amy Beeson

Amy Beeson spent her childhood in rural Staffordshire. She is a writer of fiction and non-fiction, a scriptwriter and copywriter, and runs Wordsby, a branding and communications business. Amy studied English Literature and Creative Writing at the University of East Anglia, followed by an MA in Writing and Performance for Theatre, Film and Television at the University of York. She has won prizes for poetry, has had several plays performed and was a young playwright at the Birmingham Rep where she met her husband, writer Takbir Uddin. They now live in London with their daughter, Ava.

## 1

The early autumn sun made my eyelids flutter as my brand new green Mini sped round a sharp bend at which was yet another signpost promising that the village of Totley lay a short distance ahead of me. It seemed complicit with every twist and turn of the Kent countryside to keep the hilltop village from my eagerly searching eyes. It teased me, revealing woods, then a flash of a farm at the end of a long muddy road, and the odd white weather-boarded cottage tucked away in the brambles at the edge of a copse. I was starting to feel like the place I was searching for didn't really exist; adding to my apprehension that the whole thing was a misunderstanding and when I arrived they'd tell me there had been an error and I hadn't got the job at all. After all who'd want a twenty-something health visitor straight out of training?

The road was never straight for more than a minute. I'd driven all the way from my parents' new townhouse in Staffordshire and I was desperate to be in my first home – just me, no brothers and sisters or flatmates – just me for the very first time in my life. To my great relief the raw countryside eventually gave way to high wooden gates that exposed only the numerous chimneys belonging to the big houses of the county set. And at long last a sign which read 'Welcome to Totley'. I sighed; it was beautiful and quiet and so different from the streets of Hackney – it was like arriving in another world, as my eyes delighted in the beautiful stone walls nestling cottages with bow windows and front doors separated from the pavement by only narrow porches. I felt my spirits lift and drummed along to the beat of 'Higher and Higher' by Jackie Wilson on the car radio.

The steeple of St Agatha's Church peeked out almost reticently from behind aged yew trees. As I cruised past the church a cacophony of bells rang out proudly from the belfry giving my arrival in the village a dreamlike feel. The heavy oak doors opened and wedding guests poured into the churchyard, idly nestling amongst the neglected gravestones having a quick solitary smoke or chatting in clusters of acquaintants. I looked on and smiled as the bride and groom surrounded by their closest family and friends were photographed by a man in a grey flannel suit with long sandy hair, a cigarette dangling from his lips as he forced elderly aunts in floral A-line dresses elbow to elbow with young groomsmen in stripy ill-fitting suits with yellow carnations in their buttonholes. The bride was radiant in a wide-brimmed floppy white hat and an empire-line scooped neck gown. Her dress billowed out in the breeze as she tightly held onto a small bouquet of indistinguishable pink flowers. Her bridesmaids enthusiastically tossed confetti over the happy couple, their shallow long-handled wicker baskets hung over their arms like handbags filled with yellow carnations.

I came to a crossroads and glanced down at the directions I'd scribbled when the superintendent health visitor telephoned to offer me the job:

Ivy Cottage Clinic, Main Road.
Ask Mrs Florence Farthing for keys. Next door at Primrose
    Cottage.

Main Road appeared to be the road I was on. I continued ahead and found myself in the epicentre of Totley. A row of cream cottages with brightly painted front doors faced the Village Hall and Totley Garage amongst a parade of small shops and businesses. A pair of black boots stuck out from under a Rover at the garage and multi-coloured bunting fluttered in the wind at the Village Hall, which was no doubt the venue for the wedding reception. I pulled up on the street outside the pale-blue door of Ivy Cottage at the end of the terrace. A shiny plaque told me unmistakably that it was 'Totley Clinic' – I was finally home.

I turned off the engine and jumped out of my newly acquired Mini, issued to me by 'the County' as one of the perks of the job. I'd stuffed my little car to the gunnels with the bric-à-brac and kitchenware I'd acquired during my time as a nurse in a shared flat on Balls Pond Road in London's East End; it was tilting precariously to one side. I was rather looking forward to having my own kitchen and not having to do someone else's washing-up before I could start preparing my own meal. I frowned at my school trunk which had been inexpertly strapped to the roof of my Mini by my younger brother Stephen – it was looking more dilapidated than ever. My initials 'SH' were very faded and scratched – maybe this wasn't the best first impression to give the village of their new health visitor. You must try and look older and more respectable, I scolded myself, now regretting wearing a pair of denim shorts and a white peasant blouse with delicately embroidered blue flowers to drive down in, but it was such a warm day.

Suddenly, I was worried about my appearance and took my compact out from my large brown leather handbag and inspected my face. I cleaned my black-rimmed glasses with a tissue and popped them back primly on the end of my pale-skinned nose. I bit my lips and pinched my cheeks to give myself a hint of colour and rapidly ran my fingers through my tangle of long dark hair.

Futilely I attempted to pull at the edges of my shorts towards my bare knees and cast a withering look at my raffia platform sandals looking mockingly up at me.

Taking a deep breath I knocked on the bright-yellow door of Mrs Farthing at Primrose Cottage. There was no answer. I tried again and waited a few minutes but nothing. I tried my own front door but it was locked. I could feel panic rising within me – what if there really had been a mistake and no one was expecting me at all?

My anxiety was broken by the sound of a squeak and a clanging of metal, shortly followed by the appearance of an old man with a crinkled tanned face and salt and pepper hair making his wobbly way down the street on a boneshaker of a bicycle. He was whistling to himself, completely unperturbed by the inharmonious clatter and whining of his transportation. He was balancing metal buckets on each side of the handlebars and a ladder was resting lengthways across his lap. When he saw me dawdling on the pavement outside the row of cottages his face lit up and crumpled even further at the eyes and mouth.

'Hello there, Nurse,' he called cheerily. 'She'll be out the back. We couldn't stand waiting indoors, not on such a beauty of a day.'

I smiled but didn't know what to say. Was this Mr Farthing?

He hopped nimbly off his bicycle and opened the door to the side passage. 'Follow me, Nurse,' he instructed as he took the metal buckets filled with chicken feed with him down the narrow dark tunnel. Obediently I followed. As he emerged ahead of me into the sunlight he called, 'Flo, the Nurse is here. She's arrived!'

Flo Farthing had the same tanned skin as her husband, her greying dark hair swept neatly up into a bun. She was deftly picking tomatoes from a vine, standing completely at ease in a garden filled with bed upon bed of flowers, fruit and vegetables. It's like

Mr McGregor's garden, I thought pleasantly – any minute now I will see a fat little brown rabbit popping out from a watering can. There were mature fruit trees at the back and I was sure there was a goat grazing on a stretch of pasture that ran along the end of the lane. Mrs Farthing was neat as a new pin and wore a white fitted knee-length shirt dress with green leaves and vines on it. She was diminutive and comfortingly plump, her arms and legs muscular and bronzed from a life lived outdoors. When she saw me her face lit up and she hurried towards us, hens half-flapping away at her feet, eager to get to the metal buckets of feed Mr Farthing was carrying.

I stretched out my hand and introduced myself, 'Good afternoon, Mrs Farthing. I'm Sarah Hill, the new health visitor.'

'Well, I'm very pleased to meet you, Nurse,' she gushed. 'But we'll have none of this Mr and Mrs Farthing business. I'm Flo and he's Clem. You follow me – I'll take you up to the flat and get the kettle on. As you know, Clem and I are the caretakers for the clinic. I keep it spick and span and look after you ladies, and Clem does any odd jobs that need doing. We've given your flat a good set-to this morning, haven't we, Clem?'

Clem nodded in accordance with his wife and tossed a handful of feed to the clucking hens. 'I'm going to check on Bessie.'

I looked enquiringly. 'The pig,' explained Flo. 'An Essex we got from Joe Rudcliff at Treetops Farm for fattening. And right soft Clem is about it too. Calls it Queen Bess for crying out loud.' Clem said nothing and hurried away to the pig sty at the back of their cottage garden. 'You mark my words, Clement Farthing, come Easter that porker will do very nicely indeed.' Flo's words disappeared on the cool early autumn breeze. She rearranged her face from scolding to motherly and said encouragingly, 'Follow me, dear. We'll pop in through the back gate.'

'You have a beautiful garden,' I said admiringly.

She beamed with pride. 'We've been here over 40 years. Since the day we were married.'

Flo expertly picked her way through poultry, garden produce and tools to the back lane, where the goat was thoughtfully chewing on someone else's washing line. I thought of all my belongings left unattended on the street and felt uneasy. It seemed funny to be going in through the back door.

'I think I better go back to my car and get the boxes to carry up to the flat first,' I suggested weakly.

'No need for that. Clem will do it. You don't need to lift a finger. Give me your car keys, Nurse.'

I reluctantly pulled out my precious keys from the pocket of my denim shorts. 'CLEM-eennntt,' called Flo loudly. Clem popped his head up over the garden fence. Flo chucked the keys at him without saying a word and he gave a little half-salute and scuttled off to do her bidding.

A few yards down the lane was a tatty-looking gate that stood between two enormous blackberry bushes, with a rusty catch on it. Flo struggled to open the rusty catch and gave the gate a good kick; in response it opened with a shrill squeak.

'I'll get Clem to oil that tonight,' she said more to herself than to me. 'This is the garden. You go into the clinic through the front door of the cottage. You see there's a side passage next to that little car park – well, that'll bring you from the street right to your garden. The stairs are at the back to give you a little bit of privacy.'

She tutted as we walked down the long narrow plot, past the ancient apple, pear and cherry trees, neglected vegetable patches and an abandoned greenhouse. I looked at my garden longingly. It had so much potential. This was good earth. I could save a fortune if I got it going again.

'I hope you don't think Clem and I have been neglecting our duties,' whispered Flo. 'Only Nurse Hunter, who was the old district nurse who lived in the cottage until three months back, wouldn't touch the garden. Wouldn't let us lend a hand neither. She let it go to wrack and ruin. It's criminal.'

'Oh, dear. I like gardening. Perhaps you and Clem could help me restore it to its former glory, if it's not too much trouble.'

'Would you like that, Nurse?' I nodded enthusiastically. 'It would be an absolute pleasure. I've got a good feeling about you,' she whispered conspiratorially, nudging me gently in the ribs.

'Didn't the new district nurse want the cottage?' I asked as Flo rummaged in her pockets for the keys.

'Oh, that one. She's not much older than you and she likes a good time. No, Nurse Bates didn't want to be in Totley. She turned down Ivy Cottage and opted for the bright lights of Maidstone. Wants to be near all them discotheques and swanky restaurants if you ask me.'

I quite liked the sound of Nurse Bates already. I was only in my mid-twenties; maybe I should have opted for nightlife over country life too. I'd been so thrilled to be offered the job and the flat that I hadn't really thought about how much I was giving up by moving to the sticks. Oh well, too late now, I said to myself. And I really was quite excited about my garden. I'd done plenty of going out during my Hackney days – it was time to be grown-up off-duty as well as on, I resolved.

'If you don't mind me saying, Nurse, you're the youngest health visitor I've seen – by a long way.'

I smiled. I didn't say actually the youngest in the country by all accounts.

Flo produced the keys and held them up to my face. 'Want to open the door to your new home?' she asked with a twinkle in her grey eyes. I eagerly took them off her and rattled the heavy old key in the archaic lock. Flo ceremoniously pushed open the pale-blue door with a flourish and stepped back to let me cross the threshold to my new home.

I ran up the narrow staircase, my hand running up the wooden bannisters newly painted in creamy yellow. They led straight into the kitchen and living area. It was large and bright with a window seat overlooking Main Road. It was, as Flo had said, spick and span, though a little old fashioned with frilly floral curtain covered cupboards and a beautiful old butler sink sparklingly clean. Two faded chintz armchairs were arranged neatly opposite a matching sofa and a pale-blue Formica table stood in the kitchen surrounded by bright-yellow dining chairs. On it was a box of fruit and vegetables, some milk, eggs, a loaf of bread, a packet of tea and a fruit cake next to a little vase of roses.

'Did you get these for me, Flo?' I asked, looking through the box of goodies.

'It's a little something to get you started,' she clucked.

'Thank you so much, that's incredibly kind. Let me give you some money for it,' I insisted, reaching for my purse. I was grateful for their kindness and generosity and they didn't even know me.

'Put your money away, Nurse. It's all from our garden anyway and I made the bread and the cake as today's one of my baking days, and the milk is from the cow I keep at my sister's. So, it didn't cost nothing.' Flo quickly changed the subject. 'There's a double bedroom at the back overlooking the garden,' she continued with the guided tour. 'The bathroom is through there and you'll find a little storage cupboard with a hoover and brushes in it at the end of the corridor.'

'It's lovely,' I enthused as I peeked out of the window onto the street below. Flo perched next to me on the window seat. The wedding party was now strewn around the lawn of the Village Hall. There were children running around, men drinking beer and women in floppy hats sipping wine in the sunshine. The bride and groom were greeting people as they walked past them into the hall.

'I'll have to pop over to the church soon and help the vicar tidy up – he's not married yet, bless him and he doesn't know a corn-flower from a poppy,' Flo told me.

'I hope you didn't miss the wedding on my account?' I asked.

'No, wasn't invited,' she sniffed sharply. 'His family's no better than they ought to be. Him, his brothers, his dad and his uncles all work up at the brewery and I would think they drink as much as they brew; no wonder the old place is on its way out. And she's not been in the village five minutes and her family very much keeps themselves to themselves. They're not even from Kent! Came from some town in Essex by all accounts. And you don't have to be a nurse to see you'll be visiting that girl sooner rather than later,' remarked Flo with a knowing nod.

I can't say I was salivating with the imparting of so much village gossip. I felt another short pang for city life and the anonymity of it all. Totley had looked idyllic as I drove through, but clearly life was going to be rather more sedate from now on. I sighed to myself.

The bride and groom eventually disappeared into the Village Hall after greeting the last of their guests. Flo left me to explore the rest of the flat on my own. I could hear the singing of the kettle as she prepared a little tea party to celebrate my arrival. I heard heavy footsteps running up the stairs. When I returned to the kitchen Clem was panting with his hands on his old knees as he tried to catch his breath.

'Clem, where's the nurse's belongings? What have you been doing, you old fool?' scolded Flo.

'Come quick, Nurse. Village Hall. The bride – she's not well,' puffed Clem.

I'd barely been there half an hour and was already summoned to my first medical emergency. Was this what life as a village health visitor was going to be like? I thought it would be dull compared with hospital life. How wrong I was and how glad I was to be given the wrong first impression of Totley.

Clem led me at a gallop across the street to the Village Hall. The groom and his mates had already opened a huge barrel of scrumpy and were freely pouring it into tankards from the makeshift bar. Young girls danced around their handbags in the small square of dance floor. The speakers pumped out KC and the Sunshine Band's 'Get Down Tonight'. It wasn't even five o'clock but the tranquil scene of a quiet country wedding had been transformed into a rowdy gathering of half-cut young locals. At this stage in the proceedings the youthful wedding guests were still divided into male and female, while the older crowd looked on from the sidelines – safe from speculation and free to observe in a straight row of chairs against the walls of the hall. They sat either still, their knees together sipping sherry in between tuts and the sucking in of teeth, or attempted to lounge on the uncomfortable-looking red plastic chairs while watching the heady scene wistfully, wishing they could join in with the youngsters.

Flo was hot on our heels. When we reached the back of the hall Clem stopped abruptly at the side door.

'We'll take it from here, Clem,' Flo instructed, stepping forward and relieving him of duty.

As soon as he was given a reprieve Clem scurried off back to his garden and Bessie his beloved pig. I wished I could go with him.

'What is the medical emergency?' I asked Flo under my breath.

'I would have thought that was obvious. She's having a baby.'

'Who?'

'The bride.'

'Have you called the midwife?'

'Yes, but she's in Malling, it'll take her at least half an hour to get here.'

Oh help, I thought. I'm not a midwife, I'm a health visitor and only just. Every baby I've delivered was during my obstetrics training in a hospital! I took a deep breath – I needed to take charge of the situation. This was nothing I couldn't handle. Pull yourself together, Sarah, I scolded myself. How far on can the girl be? First babies take hours and she's probably in first-stage labour or maybe even a false alarm brought on by the excitement of the wedding. Don't let your nerves get the better of you.

'Right, I'll take it from here,' I told Flo. 'Well done for calling the midwife but can you call an ambulance too. We don't want any surprises, do we?'

'Just as you say, Nurse. Give me a whistle if you need anything. I've got the keys to the clinic. I can pop in and get whatever you want until the midwife or the ambulance get here.'

'Some surgical rubber gloves and towels would be good for a start. Do you know what a foetal stethoscope is?'

'I certainly do,' Flo replied a little curtly.

'Excellent, well one of those too if you would,' I said with a broad smile. Flo was pacified.

'Righto, Nurse,' she replied, hurrying back to the clinic, glad to be of use and in the thick of it.

When I opened the door to the small cramped side room I did not find what I had been expecting; I'd imagined a slightly pink-faced bride pacing around with early labour pains. No, instead I found a frightened young woman with her dress half off, squatting between two red plastic chairs, using the seats as arm supports. An even younger bridesmaid still in her fresh buttercup gown looked pale-faced as she watched from behind the panting newlywed, whose previously neat bridal hair-do was now a tangled mess around her hot red face, her make-up smudged around her overly bright eyes.

'Hello. I'm Sarah Hill, the new health visitor,' I explained quickly and calmly, closing the door behind me.

'Thank God, you've come, Nurse. Susie Smith, I mean Bunyard. Mrs Susan Bunyard,' said the bride, panting.

'The midwife is on her way, Mrs Bunyard. But if you could put up with me until she gets here, I think we'll be able to manage between us.' She smiled briefly and then closed her eyes in preparation for the next contraction. 'When did you first start to experience labour pains?' I asked.

Susan Bunyard tried to answer me but she couldn't catch her breath. I turned my gaze towards the nervous-looking bridesmaid and smiled. The poor child couldn't have been more than 13, and she looked terrified. 'I'm Lisa. Susie's sister,' she squeaked.

'Right, Lisa. Could you go and find me a jug of water, some glasses and ice if you can,' I told her.

The girl nodded and ran out of the room, glad to be away. Flo popped her head round the door and gave me the requested equipment then tactfully retreated.

Now it was just us, I repeated my question to the expectant mother. 'When did you start to experience labour pains, Mrs Bunyard?'

'My waters broke before I put my dress on to go to church to get wed,' she said, panting, followed by a howl as she experienced a deep long contraction. I held her hand and waited for the wave of pain to be over.

'Do you mind if I take a look and see how the baby is doing?' I asked.

'Help yourself, Nurse,' she said breathlessly.

I gathered up some cushions for her to rest on the floor to give her tired arms and legs a break. Her head flopped down as she tucked herself up into a ball. I pulled on a pair of rubber gloves and scooted round to examine her.

'How many hours ago did your waters break?'

'It's only been three hours. I didn't say anything. I didn't want any delay, any excuse to postpone it. His lot would love that! I didn't want this baby born out of wedlock,' she whimpered. I could hear her breath shuddering out of her as she waited for the next contraction to come, and she didn't get to rest for long because a minute later she was gritting her teeth again.

'You're quite far on,' I said gently.

'I know, I know,' wailed the poor girl.

Lisa returned with the jugs of water and ice, and then scuttled off again.

'Do you think you could drink a little water?' I asked. She nodded and I held the glass as she took shallow sips.

'How many weeks along are you?' I asked.

'Not long enough. New Year's Eve it was. I met Aly hop picking last autumn and we got along. I knew he'd taken a shine to me. Made me promise to come to the New Year's Eve party they were having at the Brewery and, well, here we are.'

I smiled and counted in my head. 'You're 36 weeks?' I estimated. She nodded.

I hope the ambulance gets a wriggle on, I thought. Early baby coming this fast, they'd definitely need to go to Maidstone Hospital to be checked out. Steady now, Sarah, I told myself. Don't alarm her. All the possible scenarios of what could be happening were playing through my head and some of them were not good.

'The baby's almost here, isn't it?' she cried.

'Not long now,' I said softly as I held her hand.

'Oh, I can feel another contraction coming, it's a big one.' She gripped my arms as she raised herself to squat again between the two chairs and I mirrored her, doing my best to keep her safe and supported.

'Whatever happens, don't let them take the baby away, please,' she begged.

Then to my everlasting relief, the midwife appeared just in the nick of time.

'Evening, my sweetness. How far along are we then?' she asked, smiling broadly, with two dimples in her round black cheeks.

In that moment the community midwife, Ernestine Higgins, looked like an angel to me – her curvaceous figure in the doorway surrounded by a glow of light coming from the disco, crowned in her pillbox navy hat on top of her wavy bobbed black hair that had one perfect streak of white in it from the left side of her temple that ran all the way down to the back of her neck. Her navy uniform was perfectly pressed with a white starched Peter Pan collar and a thick blue belt held in place by a shiny silver buckle. The Angel Gabriel in that moment wouldn't have been a more welcome sight. The midwife shut the door and muffled the sounds of the Bay City Rollers coming from the hall.

'I'm very glad to see you, Nurse,' I told her. 'Contractions are only about a minute apart now. Mrs Bunyard's water broke only three hours ago.'

'I see. I've not seen you before have I, Mrs Bunyard?' enquired Nurse Higgins.

'No, I'm from Essex,' replied Mrs Bunyard. 'Or I was until today.'

'And is this your first baby?' asked Nurse Higgins but she didn't get a reply as Mrs Bunyard had another contraction. 'Hand me some gloves please, Nurse. Let the dog see the rabbit.' The midwife assessed the situation quickly and then picked up one of the freshly laundered towels Flo had brought over from the clinic.

'Looks like we have everything we need,' she said cheerfully. 'How are your fielding skills, Nurse?' she asked as she handed me the towel.

Her deep-brown eyes were staring intently at Mrs Bunyard's other end. I caught her eye and she nodded in confirmation.

'It's time, my sweetness,' she told Mrs Bunyard. 'The head is almost through. Next time you feel a contraction coming I want you to push into your bottom and let's get this baby out.' She'd barely got her sentence out when Mrs Bunyard screwed up her eyes and started to push. 'Quick, catch, Nurse,' called the midwife to me and there was a gush and the baby popped out. I hadn't been expecting to be holding a beautiful newborn baby in my arms on my first day in Totley, but I couldn't help but feel blessed as this tiny new life let out her first lusty cries.

'She's a wee one but there's nothing wrong with her lungs, is there?' I told Mrs Bunyard as, mesmerised, she watched her child with tears rolling down her cheeks.

Nurse Higgins sprang into action taking out all her equipment from her bag as we worked together silently and companionably, cutting the little one's cord and clearing the baby's passages. I was relieved all seemed to be well and that I hadn't forgotten my obstetrics training.

'Excellent work, ladies,' Nurse Higgins said as I placed the baby gently into the new mother's arms for the first time.

'Glad you were here ... Nurse?'

'Hill,' I replied. 'I'm the new health visitor.'

'I see,' replied the midwife. 'Good catch, by the way. Have you thought about joining the village cricket team?' She laughed. 'My husband's on the committee and they're always looking for someone in the slips.'

# 2

I tipped my half-eaten piece of toast into the bin and put my plate, cup and saucer into the sink with a rattle. Again I glanced up at the square orange clock on the wall of my kitchen; I could have sworn it was ticking more slowly than usual – how was it still only eight o'clock in the morning? I wasn't due to start at the clinic till nine; would it be bad form to be there before everyone else on my first day or show how committed I was? Come on, Sarah, no time like the present, I told myself, and decided the best option would be to locate my desk and find my way around the clinic unobserved so I wouldn't lose the whole of Monday morning working out where everything was and feeling like a postulant. Before I left I inspected myself once more in the long mirror at the top of the stairs to check I was presentable. Was my chosen ensemble of a square-necked sky-blue dress a couple of inches above the knee teamed with a cream wide-collared blouse covered in cornflowers professional enough? My shoes were smart at least thanks to my mum buying me a pair of tan-coloured pumps for a big do at Dad's work over the summer.

Pushing my black-rimmed spectacles firmly onto my nose I thought how much older I looked than on my first day as a trainee nurse, but did I really know enough to be let loose on the mothers and babies of Kent? I dearly hoped so. I thought wistfully of Daddy Davis, the charge nurse at Hackney, who'd insisted I always wear my glasses and what Sister Nivern, the harridan in charge of

Infants Ward, would say to my loose, long dark hair, free from pins and tightly wound buns. Funny how health visitors were in mufti but midwives and district nurses still had their uniforms and were recognisable in the community. When you thought about it, a health visitor on your doorstep could be anyone; the Avon lady or a well-meaning caller from the Women's Institute perhaps – but maybe that was the point?

At the front door of the clinic I rooted around in my brown leather shoulder bag for the key Flo had given me and was alarmed to discover the door was already open. I remembered in Hackney my mentor Miss Knox telling me how often the clinic there was broken into by gangs and addicts searching for drugs – but surely this wasn't the case in Totley? I crept down the chequered tiled entrance hall cursing the resounding click of my heels. Filled with uncertainty I put my hand on the handle of the first door. 'Consultation Room' was engraved on a brass sign but this door was locked. Past this was the large empty room that was used for the clinic. Grey plastic chairs were stacked against the wall behind a low table adorned with neatly piled copies of *Woman's Own* and *Horse & Hound*. A small wooden desk was pushed up against the wall and above it a poster advertising tins of baby milk. Beside it stood a couple of comfortable chairs, a set of scales, and a stack of plastic bowls and tissues on the changing tables. I pushed open another door but it was only stairs leading down to the dark cellar that served as the clinic's storeroom and I didn't fancy investigating any further down there. When I poked my head round the doors to the loo and the small kitchen a strong smell of bleach wafted at me from each. I noted that though these facilities were a bit tired and dated, like my little flat, Flo certainly kept them gleaming and in good order.

Finally, I came to the 'Health Visitors' Office' at the bottom of the corridor. The door was ajar. I peeped round the edge of the door and observed there was a desk in each of the four corners of the room and at the tidiest desk nearest the picture window sat a woman writing with a slim silver pen. A perfect line of glass vases of different shapes and sizes in pink, blue, green and yellow glass were beautifully arranged on the window sill. The coloured glass reflected the morning sunshine in a brilliant rainbow across the room. A large emerald and sapphire coloured speckled vase filled with white roses and blue and lilac freesias sat on her desk next to a collection of decorative silver photo frames. The elegant woman was wearing tortoise-shell spectacles on a gold chain round her neck, a perfectly pressed moss-green linen skirt and jacket and a violet blouse. Several rows of pea-green glass beads hung loosely round her neck as well as a gold oval-shaped locket. She was not young and must have been in her mid-forties; to me, she was the epitome of sophistication and style and not what I had expected of a country health visitor in the least. I hovered in the doorway for a few seconds watching her before she realised I was there. I couldn't help but feel a little tatty by comparison and missed the reassurance of my nurse's uniform. I nervously rocked onto the outer edges of my feet, scuffing my new shoes until a few moments later she sensed my presence. In one swift movement she immediately got to her feet while simultaneously pushing her reading glasses on top of her shiny black cropped hair to get a better look at me.

'Ah, Miss Hill, we're so glad you've come to join us,' she said warmly as she quickly walked over and ushered me in. 'Let me show you your desk. I'm Hermione Drummond.'

'It's lovely to meet you, errr' – was she a Miss or a Mrs? Oh, help, I couldn't very well call her 'Nurse'.

She immediately saw my dilemma, 'Miss Drummond. Unmarried, thank heavens,' she told me with a chuckle.

The door was nudged open with a bump and another very lofty woman stood in the doorway dressed in a burgundy polo-necked jumper and a pale-grey and brown zig-zag-patterned long skirt and cardigan. Her wavy grey hair was scooped up in large combs at the sides of her head. Unlike Miss Drummond who had a slightly bohemian air, this health visitor wore no jewellery except a gold wedding band and a three-stoned diamond ring, but she was just as smart and graceful.

I wondered if excellent deportment had been a prerequisite to health-visitor training in days gone by. Both my new colleagues were tall and filled with quiet confidence – at a little over five foot I couldn't help but feel that I didn't quite measure up in more ways than one. Stand up straight, Sarah, I told myself, stretching myself out a little more and trying to look at ease in my new surroundings. In Hackney I could be nose to chest with an outright East End gangster and not turn a hair and yet here I was inwardly quivering like a school girl. Get a grip, I told myself, as I forced my nerves down and returned their friendly smiles with a big grin of appreciation at this amiable welcome.

'Ah, Mrs King. You'll see our newest addition, Miss Hill, is with us bright and early,' Miss Drummond informed her.

Mrs King placed the wooden tray she'd been carrying onto her desk. I noted the hand-embroidered tray cloth with delicate lace edges, all laid out with a white china tea service patterned with bright green hens and foliage. Standards were clearly very high at Totley Clinic; no upturned tea chest and illicit stash of shop-bought biscuits for them.

'I had a feeling we'd see you sooner rather than later, Miss Hill,' proclaimed Mrs King with a smile. 'Hence the extra cup and saucer this morning,' she explained as she poured out the tea. There was also a stack of delicious-looking shortbread on the tray, which made my depleted appetite suddenly reappear.

'Shortbread?' she enquired. 'I made it yesterday evening while dinner was in the oven,' she told me, offering me the plate.

'Really! I had a Vesta curry on a tray in front of the telly and watched *Upstairs, Downstairs*,' I replied, astonished, and helping myself to a piece. Sarah, why did you say that, I scolded myself, shoving the shortbread into my mouth to stopper it. Homemade shortbread – my, *it was so good*.

'Oh yes, that James Bellamy is quite a dish, isn't he?' said Miss Drummond with a smile. 'Etty went to bed early and I had the place to myself. Just me, *Upstairs, Downstairs* and a large gin and tonic – one of life's lovely moments.'

'Yes, it was a good one,' agreed Mrs King. 'Even the boys watched it with Jack and me – but I don't think they'd admit it to their school friends. Then they both disappeared and camped out in the summer house all night again. I could hear Led Zeppelin drifting across the lawn until well after midnight; good job we don't have any neighbours at our place but I don't know what the hens think of it. Jack had to threaten to chuck a bucket of water over the pair of them to get them out of their sleeping bags and on time for the school bus this morning,' she said with a laugh.

'You've got two boys?' I asked.

'And a girl, Harriet, but she's at Glasgow now doing History,' answered Mrs King. 'But David and John are 15 and 17 and can let themselves in after school now, which is fine as long as the cupboards are well stocked. Teenage boys never stop eating.'

Three children, a husband and livestock to take care of *and* she works and finds a spare minute to make homemade delicacies – was she superhuman?

'Sit yourself down, Miss Hill,' instructed Miss Drummond, showing me my very own desk in the corner nearest the door.

I'd never had my own desk before and here I was at a little after eight o'clock in the morning on my very first day as a health visitor sitting in a rather swish swivel chair in front of *my* desk drinking tea and eating homemade shortbread. It was all I could do not to swirl around and around in excitement. My eyes devoured my new office space – I'd been provided with a blotter and a wicker filing tray. Brand new pens and notepads were all laid out for me, on top of which was a set of keys for my drawers. I reached into my bag and pulled out the green leather mug and letter opener I'd commandeered from my dad's desk and popped them in pride of place. I suddenly felt a little wave of importance and pleasure under-laced by the feeling I was playing at being a grown-up, with my new Mini and Ivy Cottage – what had I done to deserve any of it? I looked at my white telephone and thought any minute now there will be that call when they tell you it's all been a terrible mistake and they don't want you after all – that none of *this* is yours. But thankfully the phone didn't ring. Enjoy the moment, I told myself.

'Now you have your Mini. Did they give you a log book?' enquired Miss Drummond. I nodded. 'Good, good. Don't forget to keep your petrol receipts and mileage up to date or dear Miss Presnell will want to know why. Have you met our manager yet?'

'No,' I replied.

'She's not a bad sort. Miss Presnell doesn't bother us much does she, Mrs King?' called out Miss Drummond without pausing for a response. 'And she doesn't take too much nonsense from the top brass. Though to be honest she only comes out to the sticks on high days and holidays,' she added with a laugh. I saw Mrs King smile and arch an eyebrow at our colleague's account of our superior officer.

'And at 70 new pence to the gallon it's not a bad deal,' continued Miss Drummond. 'Where did you train?'

'Hackney,' I answered.

'Ooh, I like a girl who's trained at a proper hospital. I started out in the Wirral and then New York before I came to the Garden of England.'

'My parents lived in Sevenoaks for a few years and I went to school near Sunridge for a while.'

'You're practically a local then. You'll know your russet from your cox,' she chortled.

'We haven't got anything too gruelling for your first day. Miss Drummond and I have hearing tests at nine o'clock and I'm sorry that we'll be out for most of the day. We've got a list of your patch and a big map of the area ready, you can reconnoitre the district a bit before you hit the road,' explained Mrs King, handing me over a folder.

I eagerly opened the huge map and saw the wide expanse of countryside. 'You'll be doing Totley, the outskirts of Malling, The Meadows and the surrounding areas. At the moment that's about 800 babies and children under five plus the elderly visits we undertake.'

I looked up at her eyes wide. 'Eight hundred,' I repeated.

'And counting,' she smiled, 'not forgetting visits to the elderly to keep an eye on their general health. You're also the school nurse for St Agatha's and the Meadows Infant and Junior Schools. There's a weekly clinic in Totley but luckily for you there's only a monthly clinic run with the GP in The Meadows and at the RAF.'

'That's very fortunate,' I uttered. Eight hundred children, I thought. Eight hundred! But secretly I couldn't wait to get started. I wanted to know each one of them right now.

'So, you sit tight for today and answer the phone. You need only go out if there's an emergency,' added Miss Drummond. 'You've got your first clinic for Totley tomorrow afternoon, Mums and Toddlers on Wednesday and RAF clinic on Thursday – best you gen up on those. We'll let you loose on some clients in the middle of the week; there are a few referrals from Dr Drake, our Totley GP, to work through. His scrawls take a fair bit of deciphering, so do ask if you have any questions. All the client records for your patch are in these boxes if you need to look anything up,' she told me, tapping the two wooden index boxes already on my desk.

'Righto,' I replied. My fingers itching to get to work on the doctor's referrals and plan my week.

'And if you get a spare few minutes at lunchtime maybe toddle down to St Agatha's Primary to introduce yourself. Mr Hopkins the headmaster is very nice and Reverend Shepherd generally pops in to have lunch with the children on a Monday. It's all rather jolly,' Miss Drummond informed me as she gathered up her bag.

'Enjoy your first day,' added Mrs King. 'We'll try and pop in again in a few hours and see how you are doing. I'm sure Flo will be clucking around you anyhow.'

I'd been advised to stay put and settle in slowly and yet there I was barely an hour later lost in the Kent countryside with my sparkling Mini not just covered in mud but stuck in it. Only 20 minutes earlier I had been carefully planning out my diary for the week and making well-meant plans when my telephone tingled into life.

'Hello, Totley Clinic, health visitors,' I answered.

'Hello, Nurse?' whispered a weary voice down the line. I could hear the cries of a fractious baby in the background.

'Yes,' I responded calmly.

'Can you come out, Nurse? I've fed and fed him till I've not got a drop left. He won't stop crying, he won't go to sleep. I don't know what to do.'

'What's your name please?'

'Mandy Rudcliff.'

'And what's your baby's name and their date of birth please, Mrs Rudcliff?' I asked, my fingers already lifting the lids on the wooden boxes that contained client records – eager to get to work.

'Craig Joseph Rudcliff. I had him on 25 August.'

'Lovely, and what's your address please?'

'The Farmhouse, Treetops Farm.'

I quickly leafed through the records until I found a blank card for Craig Joseph Rudcliff; his discharge slip from Nurse Higgins had been attached with a paperclip. His primary visit was due and he was on my patch. Why not kill two birds with one stone, I decided.

'Would you like me to come out now, Mrs Rudcliff?'

'Quick as you can please, Nurse. And it's the farmhouse not the bungalow at Treetops,' she said wearily and rang off. I decided I better get to her lickety-split.

Obstructed by the quagmire I resolved there was nothing for it but to walk. I could reverse out to get back on the road to Totley but there was no way my Mini was going to make it through all that muck up the path to the farm, which I assumed was at the end of what looked like a never-ending road ascending into the clouds. I picked up my bag and swung open the door of the car and let both my feet go squelch right into the mire. Never mind the stupid map, I thought, the thing I needed right now was a good pair of wellies; from that day forth I kept a pair in the boot.

After I'd spent 10 minutes traipsing through sludge finally a house came into view. The Rudcliffs resided in a large white-washed four-storey, double-fronted Georgian farmhouse with a patch of oval-shaped lawn serving as a front garden. A fence surrounded the property creating a barrier between Treetops Farmhouse and the gargantuan tin sheds that dominated the landscape. As I trudged nearer to the house the smell coming from the pig sheds and the noise of grunting and squealing swine was overwhelming. I noticed in the distance a newly built bunga-low with a neat little garden and a border of rose bushes. It stood on top of a mound like a little castle and looked completely out of place.

I opened the gate to the farmyard and a huge hound came looming at me barking defensively. I quickly retreated and waited on the other side of the fence hoping his master would come and call him off but no one did despite all the growling and snarling from the Alsatian. I'd come this far, I wasn't going to fall at the last hurdle. 'Sit,' I said firmly, staring the animal down. To my surprise the dog obeyed so I sidestepped him and gingerly made my way to the front door and rang the bell, hoping I wouldn't be left on the doorstep too long in case my new canine friend changed his mind about me.

Mrs Rudcliff flung open the door. She was a slender woman about my height wearing a loose blue-denim shirt and jeans; she had light-brown wavy hair tied up in a ponytail and a smattering of freckles across her nose and pink cheeks. She gave me a weak smile but she looked exhausted – I suspected she was anaemic and in desperate need of sustenance and sleep. In her arms was a very robust and lengthy newborn baby; he must have been at least 10 pounds so no wonder she was finding feeding him a challenge, poor girl.

'Hello, Mrs Rudcliff?' I enquired. She nodded. 'I'm Sarah Hill, the health visitor you spoke to on the telephone.'

'Come in, Nurse,' she said. 'He only stopped crying about five minutes ago.'

I followed her down the dark hallway into the huge square kitchen. An elongated rectangular wooden table stood in its centre. At one end were bowls, spoons, a set of scales and bags of flour, all manner of ingredients, some ramekins and a fresh loaf of bread cooling on a wire rack. At the other end of the table was a heap of crumpled laundry amongst a few folded piles and two ironed shirts on hangers. An ironing board with a half-ironed shirt stood accusingly next to the table and on the floor was a basket filled with wet baby clothes, nappies, blankets and cloth squares, some of which had made it onto a clotheshorse to dry. The large butler sink in front of the kitchen window was sparklingly clean but a mountain of cups, plates and cutlery glared at us, waiting to be washed up. An enormous range stood in the hearth and before it was a button-backed tangerine sofa with an avocado throw hanging over the top.

Mrs Rudcliff looked about her in dismay. 'It was neat as a new pin a fortnight ago and now as soon as I start one job the baby needs something and nothing gets finished.'

'That's how it is for everyone,' I say softly.

'Is it?'

'Oh, yes. Between me and you, if I arrived at a house with a newborn baby that was spotless then I'd be concerned.'

She laughed a little in relief. 'Sit yourself down, Nurse. I'll make us some tea.'

'Would you let me make it? Take the weight off your feet for five minutes,' I gently suggested.

'Are you sure?' I nodded and she flopped onto the sofa and closed her eyes for a few minutes with the baby lying happily across her chest while I put the kettle on. I brought over the tea with a large glass of water and a plate of biscuits I'd seen on the side.

'Would you let me have a hold of baby Craig?' I asked as I set down the tea things on a small side table.

'Be my guest,' replied Mrs Rudcliff, handing over her whopper of a baby. The tea, water and biscuits had all vanished within minutes and it gave me the chance to give the baby a quick once-over. 'I'm always hungry at the moment,' she told me, flicking crumbs off her shirt.

'It's the breastfeeding,' I acknowledged. 'You need plenty of good food and lots to drink to sustain both you and the baby.'

She sighed. 'I only get the chance to grab a quick piece of toast these days and a cold cup of tea if I'm lucky. As soon as I put the dinner on the table the baby cries and by the time I come back it's either stone cold or Joe's given it to the dog.'

'I bet you have a job just making the dinner,' I said, pouring her another cup of tea and refilling the biscuits.

'I do, I do. I can barely get myself washed and dressed by lunchtime. And the men expect a hot meal at breakfast, lunch and dinner.'

'It's you who needs a good dinner three times a day and snacks in between.'

'Do you think so?'

'Absolutely. Also try and have a glass of water next to you while you're feeding and have a glass to sip throughout the day and night.'

'I'll try. It's so hard to get everything together when he's crying for a feed.'

'I know it seems like a lot but you need all those little drinks and snacks to make the milk. It'll do him no harm to wait two minutes while you get a cuppa and a snack and pop to the loo. You'll be able to feed better for it.'

'I can't tell you how many times I'm been bursting to go to the loo during a feed. I've near wet myself at least twice this morning. I thought it would make me a bad mum if I didn't run to him straight away. When he cries my heart pounds like crazy.'

'That's perfectly normal. You have some basic needs too; it's not asking much that you get the chance to eat, drink and wash, is it?'

'I guess not.'

'Try and stick to two or three cups of tea or coffee a day, as the caffeine can make the baby restless. If you have a nice milky malted drink before bedtime it might help him doze off a little easier.'

'Right. I hadn't thought of that. I was drinking all that tea and coffee to help me stay awake – I didn't realise it would have the same effect on him.'

'Not to worry. I can't think straight in the morning until I've had a cup of tea and I don't have a newborn baby keeping me up.'

'Or a husband snoring in your ear when the baby goes down and you get a chance for forty winks?' she said, giggling.

'No,' I agreed, with a chuckle. 'Fortunately not. Do you think Mr Rudcliff could help with the housework and cooking a bit?' I suggested.

She looked me straight in the eye and said, 'No, Nurse. He's a male chauvinist pig farmer,' and we both burst out laughing for at least a minute.

'Do you have any family nearby who could help?' I asked.

'My mum's in Cheltenham. I don't like to bother her.'

'Has she offered to help?'

'Lots of times but I don't want her to think I can't cope. I want her to be proud of me; she always had everything immaculate when I was little and look at this place!' she said, casting her eyes round the farmhouse kitchen in dismay.

'Housework always needs doing. I don't see the harm in letting things slide for a little while.'

'Oh! My mother-in-law said you'd be coming to see I kept the place clean and tidy or you'd report me.'

'Not at all,' I told her. 'Are your husband's family able to lend a hand?'

'His parents live in the bungalow. Did you see it on your way in?'

'Yes, up on the mound?'

'Ghastly, isn't it? I wouldn't ask his mother to help me in a month of Sundays. She'd love nothing better than to get back into

28

the farmhouse kitchen and shove me out. I won't have it,' she told me, getting quite worked up. Baby Craig started crying again.

'I've only just fed him. Really I have,' she said, her voice fading and her eyes glazing over.

'Long babies can be difficult to feed,' I explained.

'Can they?'

'Yes, and he was 10 pounds and six ounces when he was born and I can see from his discharge papers he's nearly made his birth weight up already. That means you're doing a fantastic job,' I soothed.

'I'm finding him a bit heavy. He's only two weeks old and he's already a handful – how am I going to cope?' she asked as tears started to trickle down her freckled cheeks and her narrow shoulders shook as she took short intakes of breath. 'I feel so lost sometimes. One minute I'm looking at him and my heart is fit to burst, I love him so much. But there are times in the middle of the night when I feel utterly alone. Joe's snoring, none the wiser, the baby won't go down in his crib and I'm so tired I can barely see straight. I swear I've seen the sunrise every morning since Craig was born.' I sat by her side and listened, nodding and acknowledging her feelings. 'Why did no one tell me it would be this hard? I don't recognise myself at the moment and Joe's life carries on exactly the same.'

'Let's look at one thing at a time. You're doing really well, Mrs Rudcliff, you really are. What do you think could be better?'

'The feeding. He's so heavy, and he pounds on me with his fist and thrashes about and leaves me aching. I dread it, I really do, and it's not getting any easier. I'm not fit to be his mother.'

'You are a splendid mother. Do you think an unfit mother would care this much?'

She gave me a little shy smile. 'I suppose that's right. You'd know, Nurse.'

An hour later Craig was sleeping peacefully, we'd discussed feeding, sleeping and nappies, and Mrs Rudcliff was calmer but I was still worried about her health. She needed a bit of looking after. The kitchen door swung open and Joe Rudcliff appeared. A burly man and at over six feet his head practically scraped the ceiling as he came in. Silently he pulled off his muddy boots and went to wash his hands and face in the kitchen sink. He didn't say a word or even show the slightest awareness there was a stranger, *me*, in his house.

'What's for lunch?' he asked his wife, his back to us as he gazed out of the kitchen window onto his empire.

'I've made mackerel pâté and freshly baked bread.'

'Again?'

She nodded.

'I'll be half-starved in a month if you carry on this way,' he informed her, taking a huge hunk of bread from the kitchen table and spreading it liberally with the delicious looking pâté. He stomped off, followed a minute later by the sound of the radio blaring from the sitting room.

'I'm going to go now if there isn't anything else?' I asked. But Mrs Rudcliff didn't reply. 'While the baby's asleep eat up some of that scrumptious pâté and then get your head down for a bit if you can.'

'Would you like some?'

'No, thank you. You eat it all up while you can.'

'I will, Nurse,' she said. A tone of defiance creeping into her voice. 'But before that I'm going to telephone my mother and see if she can come for a bit.'

'I think that's an excellent idea, Mrs Rudcliff. I'll call in next week and see how you are but do telephone me at the clinic if you need anything.'

As I made my way back down the path to my abandoned Mini

I turned and saw Mrs Rudcliff in the window with a telephone in her hand. I grinned. Good for you, I thought. My first visit as a health visitor had been a good one but what did the other 799 and counting have in store?

When I returned to see Mrs Rudcliff at Treetops Farm the following week I fully prepared for the ascent in a pair of newly acquired black Wellington boots purchased at a smart little shop in Canterbury. I'd christened them on my second Sunday in Kent, digging over my small vegetable patch after borrowing a fork and spade from Clem. It would be a while before I could sow anything but at least I'd made a start – I was well on my way to becoming a country nurse, or so I thought.

# 3

I knew I was frowning slightly as Flo poured me a cup of tea before the doors opened for the two o'clock Totley baby clinic on Tuesday afternoon. I'd been stunned when Mrs Martha Bunyard, a matriarch of clinic volunteers, had practically shoved me into the cramped consulting room away from the hall when I arrived, but now I was fuming.

'Your predecessor always saw mothers in here, Nurse. That's the way we've always done it in Totley. Stops time-wasters taking liberties,' she had informed me.

We'll see, I thought as I agitatedly sipped my tea. Flo looked at me thoughtfully. 'Don't want to rock the boat at your very first clinic, do you?' she suggested tentatively. 'Martha Bunyard and Doris Bowyer have been running things round here for years, Nurse. No one likes change, do they?'

'Hmm,' I replied. I thought of Susan, whose baby I'd helped deliver only days before, and felt a pang of sympathy for her. The stalwart so-called helper, who was most likely banking on me being out of sight and out of mind, was probably a relative of Susan's new husband, his mother even – poor girl.

Flo straightened the biscuits on her trolley. 'Have you got through that vegetable box we left you, yet?' she asked, changing the subject.

'Still working my way through it. Best produce I've ever tasted,' I enthused.

Flo beamed with pride. 'I don't like to boast but my Clem has won "Best in Show" for his root vegetables at the village fete every single year for the last decade. Beetroot, carrot, potato, you name it, he's won the blue ribbon for it. Mr Hopkins and Father Nick are almost green with ...' She stopped herself. 'Pride comes before a fall,' she reminded herself. 'Lots to do; while you're all out and about I think I'll give the health visitors' room a quick once over with a duster,' she muttered to herself. 'Mrs Drummond does have rather a lot of knick-knacks that are magnets for dust,' she added, bustling off behind her tea trolley. 'And Mrs Jefferies is in today. She'll be running a gloved finger over everything, you mark my words.'

Oh yes, I still had to meet the fourth health visitor; 'Mrs N. Jefferies' read the little name plaque she had facing outwards on her desk. I scowled again at the thought of Mrs Martha Bunyard telling me what to do. Maybe I'd needed to be firmer from the off? I must stop sulking, I decided. I needed to observe and see how it all went. If it worked for the mothers then it didn't matter if I was shut away in the dreary claustrophobic backroom.

There was a tap on the semi-open door. I saw a woman in a yellow and cream V-necked floral dress with tiny round buttons plus matching russet jacket and sandals standing in the doorway. Her almost white blonde hair was pulled off her face by a couple of golden combs. Her eyes wrinkled into deep furrowed lines as she gave me a broad open smile.

'Knock, knock,' she called as she stepped into the room. 'I thought I'd come and say hello. I'm Monika Michalak, the clinic doctor.'

'Where have they shut you away?' I asked, stepping forward. 'Sorry,' I corrected myself, realising how much I was giving away, 'I'm Sarah Hill, the new health visitor.'

'Don't worry. They do rather like to tuck us out of harm's way in the broom cupboard, don't they?' she said, laughing. 'I turn up and do my bit. But I often think it's a shame we only see a mother by request.'

I smiled thoughtfully, drinking in the situation. Wait and see, wait and see, Sarah, don't be too hasty, I said to myself.

Dr Michalak cast her eyes down, smiling shyly as she checked her wristwatch. 'Doors open in a minute – action stations,' she said merrily as she slipped away, back to her own closet.

Half an hour later and there I was drumming my fingers on the desk not having seen a single soul. Had nobody come yet? As a student health visitor I'd never been to a clinic that wasn't packed right from the off. Maybe people didn't go to clinic here; had I come to somewhere that had no need for me? 'I'm not spending every Tuesday afternoon twiddling my thumbs. I'm going to go out there to see for myself what's going on.' I gingerly made my way to the main reception. Three of the four clinic volunteers were in a little huddle in a closed circle of chairs having cups of tea and biscuits in a corner; Mrs Martha Bunyard was very much the Queen Bee. Toddlers were running around or whining hot and bored with nothing to do. At least one of them was doing something helpful by weighing the babies, albeit fully clothed. None of the changing tables had been set up and chairs for the mothers to sit on seemed to be very few and far between. 'It's not good enough,' I fumed.

'Any mothers waiting to be seen?' I asked my so-called volunteers.

'What you doing out here, Nurse?' replied Mrs Martha Bunyard in an accusatory tone. 'We'll tell you if anyone wants you.' And before I knew it I was back in my box. I only saw three mothers during the clinic and felt utterly useless. I glumly trudged back to the office to see if there'd been any messages – probably not; maybe the mothers didn't want to see me? As I shuffled past the clinic room I overheard Mrs Martha Bunyard saying, 'Slip of a girl, barely a nurse. What does she know about babies and motherhood that we don't?'

Fuming, I marched up to her and made a declaration of war. 'I'll have the clinic keys from now on please, Mrs Bunyard.'

She gaped at me for a few moments before replying, 'I've had these keys for 30 years.'

'Well, they'll be perfectly safe with me.'

'What do you need them for?'

'It'll give me the opportunity to set up the clinic in a new way. Next week I'd like you to come 10 minutes beforehand and I'll run through the changes with you all.'

'We've been doing this clinic like this for decades.'

'Times change.'

'Not in Totley.'

'The keys please, Mrs Bunyard.'

Reluctantly she opened her handbag. 'They'd be much safer with me. You won't lose them, will you? I've had this same set since 1945.'

'I'm perfectly capable of looking after a pair of keys, Mrs Bunyard.'

She frowned. 'The silvery one is for the toy cupboard.'

'Thank you.' Not that they'd bothered to put any toys out in the first place.

'And the brass one is for the metal cupboard where we keep the baby milk and whatnot.'

'That seems simple enough,' I said, smiling through my teeth as I took the keys out of her grasping hand and sauntered off back to my desk, leaving a buzz of whispered outrages behind me.

A plump woman with grey hair pulled back off her round face highlighting a bulbous red nose was blocking the entrance to the health visitors' office. She wore a long plain tweed skirt teamed with a tightly buttoned dusty brown shirt. She was clearly leaving as her alligator handbag was securely nestled in the crook of her arm, car keys already in hand, balancing a large tin of what looked like Mrs King's homemade shortbread biscuits and a stack of files underneath it.

'Hello, I'm Sarah Hill, the new health visitor,' I greeted her.

'I don't have time for pleasantries, but as you're here you can make yourself useful and carry these to my car,' she said, giving me the wad of records but keeping tight hold of the biscuits.

I followed her in silence out of the clinic to the car park, where she plonked everything on the backseat of her own Mini.

'My, my! I would have thought you a student nurse on community practice at first glance,' she remarked, her eyes cast down at my short skirt. 'When I trained nurses wore skirts a good four inches below the knee on and off-duty.'

I wanted to ask if that had been during the Crimean War but I bit my lip.

'Are you finished for the day, Mrs Jefferies?' I asked. It was only four o'clock and I knew Mrs King and Miss Drummond would be back soon to write up their notes.

'I am, but I don't see what business it is of yours.'

I didn't know what to say. She got into the driver's seat of her car. 'I'll see you tomorrow, Mrs Jefferies,' I said, attempting cheeriness.

'You will not. I only come to Totley Clinic on Tuesdays and Thursdays.'

'Oh, are you part-time?' I asked innocently.

Her eyes burned into me. 'I work from the doctors' surgery in Malling the rest of the week. I do not visit farm workers and villagers. Totley is not under my jurisdiction I am happy to say.

They are entirely in your hands, Miss Hill. Good afternoon,' she ticked me off before slamming her car door on me.

I scowled as I forlornly watched Mrs Jefferies speed off in a cloud of dust. They certainly make the women thorny in these parts, I ruminated, agitatedly flicking Mrs Martha Bunyard's precious keys back and forth in my hand. I had notes to write up but what with overbearing volunteers at clinic and now, to top it all, it being clear that Mrs N. Jefferies had taken a distinct dislike to me on first sight, I started to feel perhaps moving to Totley had been a terrible mistake. I flicked the keys faster and faster, back and forth, biting my lower lip, and then somehow the keys slipped out my hand and down the drain of the clinic car park. 'Oh hell, that woman had those keys for 30 years and I'd not had them for 10 minutes and look at what I've done,' I lamented, getting onto my hands and knees to see if there was any way to retrieve them from the drain. What a mess!

I must have looked a sorry state when Miss Drummond gracefully entered the room. She dropped her bag onto a chair and sat on the edge of her desk, smiling curiously at me, my hair a-tangle, with smudges of clinic car-park dust on my face and clothes.

'How was your first clinic, Miss Hill?' she asked.

'All right,' I responded, attempting nonchalance.

'I hear waves were made and the tables turned,' she remarked, a smile playing on her lips.

I stared at her blankly then blurted out, 'I dropped Mrs Bunyard's keys down the drain.'

'Oh dear. What are you going to do about that?'

'Look for another job?'

'No.'

'Eat humble pie.'

'A bit bitter for my taste, Miss Hill.'

'What then?'

'Do you think they're the only keys? I'm sure Mrs Farthing could get you a new pair cut if you ask her nicely.'

'Miss Drummond, you're a genius.' Now, I had to figure out how I was going to turn around the clinic so I wasn't relegated to the back room – but I had a week to come up with a plan.

'Anything to put a smile back on that forlorn-looking face. But you're still frowning?'

'I met Mrs Jefferies,' I mumbled.

'Ah,' sympathised Miss Drummond. 'I wouldn't take it to heart. She's never liked Totley. She was the health visitor here many moons ago. Unfortunate to be the school nurse with a name like Nora. She took offence her very first week so quickly found a role visiting the gentry in Malling and of course she's completely enamoured of the doctors there – much more well-to-do. She's very stuck in her ways. Whatever she says, remember, she always needs a saucer of cream afterwards.'

I laughed with relief. It wasn't just me. Mrs Jefferies was clearly a complete cat to everyone as Miss Drummond had cleverly pointed out.

Miss Drummond shrugged off a long crimson shawl she'd been wearing and opened up a cupboard and took out a bottle of sherry and two glasses.

'Mrs King keeps a bottle of sherry to spice up her soup at lunchtime but the sun is over the yardarm, so let's call it a day and have a drink,' she said, pouring each of us a glass. 'It's a beautiful September evening. Why don't we have them in your little garden?' she suggested. 'If that's not too presumptuous of me?'

'No, no, I think that's a lovely idea,' I said, quickly gathering up my things and rising to my feet.

Miss Drummond followed me round to the back of the clinic and through the back gate into my long garden. Over the fence

Clem and Flo were hard at work. Flo was picking ripe tomatoes and Clem was in his element in his white beekeeper's suit.

'A very devoted couple,' remarked Miss Drummond.

'They've been very kind,' I added.

Miss Drummond caught Clem's eye and he edged away from the hives, lifting the net off his hood.

'Evening, ladies,' he called. 'I'm harvesting my honey.'

'Best honey in the whole county,' praised Miss Drummond.

'I don't know about that,' mumbled Clem, glowing with pleasure. 'But I'll make sure I keep at least half a dozen jars for each of you when I've finished heeving.'

'You're too kind, Clem.'

'Getting ready for winter, Clem?' I asked.

'I am, Nurse. Got to make sure there's at least 60 pounds of sugar to keep the bees going or the queen won't have it.'

'Giving them plenty of syrup too?' I asked.

Clem raised his eyes in surprise. 'I am, Nurse, as it goes.'

I smiled. 'My father comes from a long line of beekeepers,' I explained.

'And does he have his own heeves?'

'He does. My parents are living in the town now, but he still keeps a hive or two at the bottom of their garden and more with a farmer nearby.'

'Maybe we could set you up with a little heeve of your own,' he suggested.

'I don't think I'm ready for that. But I'd gladly help you,' I offered.

'Clement, let the ladies alone,' Flo called across the garden. 'They've had a hard day, they don't want to listen to you droning on about your bees all evening. It's bad enough I have to listen to it.'

'Ah, Mrs Farthing, just the woman we need,' coaxed Miss Drummond. 'Miss Hill is in need of a fresh set of keys for the clinic including the store cupboards – do you think you could get some cut for her?'

'No trouble at all, Miss Drummond. I'll get onto it first thing tomorrow.'

'You're a treasure, Mrs Farthing.'

'Thank you so much,' I gushed. To think only an hour before I'd felt like jumping in my Mini and fleeing Totley for ever.

Clem smiled and returned to his frames, Flo to her tomatoes, and Miss Drummond and I dusted off the little table and chairs by my back door and settled down with our sherry.

'So, you're a country girl?' remarked Miss Drummond.

I nodded. 'Did you grow up in Kent?'

'Lord, no. Edinburgh. We've been here for the last 10 years ever since I came back from New York.'

'I see,' I answered, but I didn't at all.

'How are you finding the flat?'

'It's lovely. I've got everything I need.'

'Well, that's a blessing.'

'Do you live in the village, Miss Drummond?'

'Please call me Hermione off-duty, and may I call you Sarah?' I nodded and she smiled. 'We have a little cottage down by the river on Mill Lane.'

'Oh, how lovely.'

'It suits us – you must come and see us sometime?' said Hermione, as she sat back, closed her eyes and bathed in evening sunlight. 'You know the previous occupant of Ivy Cottage was the old district nurse? She left us only two months ago.'

'Flo mentioned it. She said the new district nurse had opted to live in Maidstone and turned down the flat.'

'Yes, Miss Bates. Pretty girl. Full of gusto. I'm sure you'll get on. Did Flo happen to mention where the old district nurse moved to?'

'No, she didn't.'

'Hove.'

'Near Brighton?'

'Yes,' she paused and opened one eye momentarily for dramatic effect, 'with Mr Jefferies.'

My eyes widened. 'I'd assumed she'd retired. You mean the husband of …?' My words trailed off.

'Indeed, you can see why our colleague is feeling anti-sex appeal?'

I nodded. I felt quite sorry for Mrs Jefferies. No wonder she'd rolled her eyes at my hemlines. I wondered if they'd been carrying on in my flat.

'Another reason for her to loathe Totley,' explained Hermione, opening her eyes momentarily. 'Apparently, he used to come over Monday, Wednesday, Friday …'

'… and Mrs Jefferies works at the clinic on Tuesdays and Thursdays,' I finished.

She nodded. 'Rumour has it, that it all started at last year's staff Christmas party, and in a small village Mr Jefferies regularly stopping by the clinic, or Ivy Cottage more likely, was bound to be noticed.' Hermione took a long sip of her sherry as I waited to hear more. 'I remember them running away together well because Billie Jean King was thrashing Evonne what's-her-name in the Wimbledon final and they scarpered while everyone was engrossed in the match. Proved to be a bit of an anti-climax really.'

'The affair?'

Hermione giggled. 'No, the match. It was all over in no time.' And then she raised an eyebrow to wordlessly finish off the account.

I chuckled. 'And what does Mrs Jefferies say about it?'

'Oh, nothing at all,' Hermione elaborated, her sherry finished. 'She never alludes to the affair and if pressed will confide she showed him the door after discovering some troubling things in his genealogy or some such rubbish.'

'She sounds like a snob.'

'We're all snobs, Sarah, it's a question of degree.' I smiled. She was right of course. 'Now, I really must be getting back to Etty. It's long past dinnertime. Enjoy the rest of your evening. Anything exciting planned?'

'No, nothing at all,' I sighed with a little pang for London life. When you lived with other nurses in the metropolis there was always something to do, someone to pal up with. I suddenly felt very alone.

'I've always rather enjoyed my own company,' Hermione told me as if she'd read my thoughts. 'No one to boss you about. You can lie down, have a nice cocktail and enjoy a good book, a bubble bath or something jolly on the radio without asking anyone's permission. I often look at young girls rushing off to the altar and think it's such a shame, why can't they have a bit of freedom? God knows for most of our sex the opportunities for self-indulgence are few and far between. Enjoy it while you can,' Hermione advised sagely with a wink before she sauntered off down the garden path.

# 4

My second week in Totley began with a visit to the doctor. If you were feeling chipper when you entered the village surgery it was unlikely you'd still be bright and breezy when you departed. I eyed up the receptionist behind the desk wearily. I'd only popped in to ask Dr Drake about a referral he'd given me for an old lady, and didn't appreciate being told to sit there like a lemon for half an hour. He'd seen all his patients, and the Victorian oak-panelled waiting room with its arsenic green peeling paint had been completely vacant of another soul for the last 10 minutes. As I watched the receptionist's fake-pink fingernails slowly tap away on her typewriter as she ignored the ringing telephone I felt increasing narked. I didn't believe she'd even told Dr Drake I was waiting – I think she was one of those sadistic doctors' receptionists who stick their noses into people's business and think they're one down from a physician and gossip about you behind your back.

A thin man with greased-back black hair lurched out of a consulting room. His suit looked older than he was and had been pressed until it was practically threadbare. He looked about 40-odd. His eyes were narrow and his nose red. He ignored me completely and tip-toed over to the receptionist's desk until he was right behind her.

'Miss Barrow,' he wheezed into her ear.

She jumped with surprise and broke off one of her ghastly nails on the typewriter. She yelped and looked up at him with wide doe-eyes. He took the damaged finger in his hand and looked it over carefully.

'You'll live,' he told her curtly, dropping her limp hand. 'Pop back to the kitchen at the house and get me a bacon sandwich, would you? I'm absolutely ravenous.'

'Yes, Dr Botten,' she gasped. I dropped my shoulders with relief; this wasn't Dr Drake – I hadn't been wasting my time waiting for *him* at least.

'Oh, and be a good sport and give my golf clubs a polish while you're there. I've got a game this afternoon with Captain Beauchamp-Smith and we wouldn't want me letting the side down, would we? I plan to thrash him and then drink him under the table at the nineteenth hole up at the new course on Fairy Hill.'

'Certainly, Doctor. I was planning on popping back anyway. There's all the laundry to catch up on.'

'Yes, no slacking now,' Dr Botten replied, wagging his finger and then staggering back to his room, still without casting a single look in my direction.

I didn't like the cut of his jib. I almost felt sorry for Miss Barrow, his besotted receptionist-cum-housekeeper. Clearly a slave driver and I bet he paid a pittance looking at the state of the décor in his surgery and his suit.

With no one on guard, I decided to take matters into my own hands and tapped on Dr Drake's door. I knocked and heard a not unfamiliar sound. Not so much a reply but a low mumbling noise. Typical doctor too lofty to even call 'Come in', I thought as I rolled my eyes and pushed open the heavy door. Dr Drake was sitting in his chair in front of his battered old desk, eyes closed, head dropped onto his chest. He looked dead to the world. I peered at him; I hope he hasn't kicked the bucket, I thought, edging closer. Then with relief I noticed the rise and fall of his chest. His lips were slowly parted and a long slow deep humming noise seeped out as he exhaled.

'Dr Drake,' I squeaked.

He kept his eyes shut and briefly raised one hand to silence me. I waited a few moments and took the opportunity to study him more closely. He was way past retirement age, I'd say nearer 70 than 60; maybe he needed a nap after an exhausting morning's surgery. He let out a loud long breath, lifted his head up then opened his bright eyes and smiled at me.

'Are you our new nurse?' he enquired, warmly rising to his feet.

'Yes, I'm Sarah Hill, the new health visitor.'

He shook my hand gently. His skin was soft and papery. 'A pleasure to meet you, Nurse Hill. Forgive me for keeping you on tenterhooks but between the hours of 9.55 and 10.15 in the morning I practice Transcendental Meditation and am never to be disturbed unless it is an absolute emergency. Did Miss Barrow not explain that?' I shook my head. 'Ah, well now you know. It's been my habit to meditate morning and afternoon since the war. Before the war I used to let off steam with a round of golf, but since I discovered the art of meditation I haven't picked up a club. Gave them lock, stock and mashie niblick to Dr Botten's father, my former partner.'

'Yes, I expect they are still in good use.'

'You may be right. Have you studied relaxation, Nurse Hill?'

'I haven't, no.'

'I cannot recommend it enough. I discovered it rather late in life. I was a man of 50 when I first saw the gurus in India talk about the expansion of happiness and the power of the concentrated mind during my somewhat semi-active duty there in the war.'

I did a quick calculation in my head. Surely he wasn't over 80? My goodness – maybe there was something in this Transcendental Meditation lark.

'What are the benefits, Doctor?' I asked.

'Relaxation, the reduction of stress, a space for a positive sense of self and I would say the connection to one's spiritual inner-being. As a GP I treat the body, but as you may have experienced healing is often as much to do with our state of mind. I can't write out a script for that.'

'Yes, I know what you mean. Sometimes, with the mothers I've often thought it's the anxiety they're experiencing that contributes towards issues for themselves and their babies.'

'How very perceptive of you, Nurse.'

'Though, I think they would struggle to find 15 minutes of uninterrupted time to meditate twice a day.'

'You may be right,' he chuckled.

I returned to the purpose of my visit. 'Doctor, you've sent me a request to call on an elderly lady, a Mrs Wimble who lives at Peasblossom.'

'I have, yes.'

'Is there a particular ailment that you want me to address during the visit?'

'I haven't the foggiest, Nurse Hill.'

'I'm sorry. Why have you requested a home visit? I don't mind but I wouldn't want to step on the district nurse's toes.'

'Neither Nurse Bates nor I can get so much as a toe in the door. Mrs Wimble refuses to attend the surgery and we've both failed to make it over the parapet at her camp. I've brought in the reserves.'

'Me?'

'Yes, you, Nurse Hill. If you aren't able to make the old battle-axe see sense then I'm afraid I will have to refer her to the big guns.'

'You mean the Welfare Department?'

'Indeed. And judging by the outward appearance of that tumbledown cottage of hers I think it unlikely they would allow Mrs Wimble to remain in her own home.'

'And I'm guessing Mrs Wimble would hate that?'

'Exactly so. I can't see her keeping on in a sanitised nursing home for even a month. The mind often takes root, and Mrs Wimble is definitely an ancient oak.'

'I'll call on her this afternoon, Doctor.'

'Good luck. You're our last hope.'

I smiled and slipped out.

That afternoon I ventured in my green Mini up and down the rolling hills of Totley en route to Mrs Wimble's on the very outskirts of the village. I switched on the radio, heard a single line of 'In the Summer Time' and twiddled the dial pretty sharpish to change stations and discovered my old favourite tune 'Yellow River'. I sang along to drown out thoughts of Hackney and my ex-boyfriend and the memories of previous summers that Mungo Jerry had inadvertently conjured up.

Soon the neat rows of terraced stone houses gave way to large detached and gated abodes, and then to copses and weather-beaten boarded cottages that stood on the edges of little hop gardens or orchards. Every smallholding and hedgerow seemed full of people beginning to reap the fruits of their labour: apples, pears, plums and of course beer. I almost wished I could take the afternoon off and be out in the September sunshine with them until my bucolic reveries were interrupted by a speeding van from Totley Brewery forcing me to swerve into a ditch. I recognised the driver in his brown overalls and rolled-up sleeves sitting high up in the van, oblivious to the oncoming traffic. The last time I'd seen him he'd been grinning like the Cheshire Cat, slightly the worse for drink in a grey beer-stained suit holding his newborn baby girl. I'd been worried he'd drop his bundle of joy but he thankfully proved me wrong. It was Alan Bunyard, and I'd be doing the primary visit for his wife Susan next week. Before I had a chance to curse him he was already out of sight in my rear-view mirror. Ah well, no harm done, I told myself as I shakily restarted the engine and continued on my journey.

The close encounter left me feeling tense and it was no surprise that I drove straight past the narrow almost indistinguishable lane that led to Mrs Wimble's cottage and had to reverse back up the road. Squinting in the late afternoon sun at the faded wooden sign hanging on a rusty chain across the driveway I made out the name of the smallholding: Peasblossom. Well, that's the one! Hermione had said the house was in a corner of Fairy Woods over the hills. I jumped out and unclipped the stiff latch attached to a decaying wooden post which was thick with late-blooming dill and mugwort in a plush carpet at its base. Once through I couldn't be bothered to get out of the car again and decided to leave the entrance open for the time being and put the chain back on when I left, uncertain of how much of a deterrent this was. Later, I came to wonder if it had been Mrs Wimble who had marked her property as out of bounds or some other person.

As I trundled up the narrow driveway, acres of tall grass tangled with weeds and wildflowers towered on each side, gently brushing the roof of my Mini as we slowly passed by. Ancient chestnut, hazel and willow trees lined the road and behind them was a dense wood of beeches and oaks casting huge shadows on the sunlit lane. I turned off my radio and wound the window down. The woods seemed alive; the buzzing, fluttering and shuffling of creatures created a mellow hum that remained steady under the high-pitched rustle of the wind through the leaves. Those high branches were home to calling chiffchaffs and nightingales, a fuzzy mix of yellows and browns to the naked eye but their song was delightfully distinct. I thought momentarily of a childhood summer holiday and my dad reading me passages of H.E. Bates on the beach in Sandgate while my siblings clambered over rocks with their buckets, nets and raw knees, and felt warmed by this distant memory of ice creams, shrimping and most of all reading his books. In my little flat in Totley a well-loved copy of *The Darling Buds of May* waited on my bedside table and a pang for a family of my own went through me for a moment. I pushed it down; it wasn't on my path just yet.

The lane stopped short of Mrs Wimble's house, if you could call it a house. One side seemed to have collapsed completely and heaps of rotting boards lay in piles in the farmyard. Creeping plants obscured the rooms from outside view at every sooty window. A black cat ran straight in front of my car, forcing me to screech to a halt. She gave me a disdainful look as she ran across my path, a live mouse clenched in her jaws and a litter of mewing mahogany and ebony kittens running behind her. I looked at the muddy farmyard busy with ducks, geese and chickens and retrieved my wellies from the boot of the car.

As I opened the gate and ventured down the garden path a flapping of wings was visible in the corner of my eye before my ears were assaulted with a terrifying honk as a snow-white gander charged me. No use telling this one to sit, I thought, as I ran to the door and attempted to bat him back with my large diary and called out for dear life for Mrs Wimble to open the door, but there was no reply. Eager to be away from this awful creature that any second now was going to do me a serious mischief, I ran round the side of the house with the gander hot on my heels and found the kitchen door open. I brushed him back with a besom broom and shut the kitchen door right in the horrid bird's beak as he continued to honk and flap angrily outside. He's fiercer than any guard dog, I thought.

Before I saw the squalor of Mrs Wimble's kitchen I smelt it. Cat wee and, worse, decomposing scraps of food, dust and smuts formed a film on every surface. Moggies sitting in the sink and on the table, which was covered in soil, fauna and flora as well as dirty plates and crusted cups. The Baby Belling oven housed a mother cat and her kittens not to mention the abandoned range, which appeared for all intents and purposes to be a feline hotel. I held my nose and called once more for Mrs Wimble but there was still no answer. Cautiously I made my way out of the kitchen and down the hallway, which was lined with piles of newspapers, books and more plants.

In the parlour I spotted a tall black fur hat over a high-backed faded blue armchair spotted with holes in the upholstery. Baskets of wool encircled this disintegrating throne and I was surprised to find beautifully knitted unblemished garments strewn on every stick of worm-infested furniture.

'Mrs Wimble?' I called softly once more.

In front of the old lady crowned in her black hat was a spinning wheel. She looked like something out of the Brothers Grimm as she slumbered majestically, ragged and alone in a forgotten house. Mrs Wimble was dressed in damask dressing gown with a discoloured golden cord tied around her shrinking waist and instead of carpet slippers she too wore Wellington boots. For the second time that day I was filled with the horror that I'd discovered a dead body. I edged closer and felt for a pulse and the old lady juddered into life as she felt the coldness of my hand on her carotid artery.

'And who are you?' she hissed, peering at me through the gloom.

'I'm Sarah Hill, the new health visitor. Dr Drake asked me to call on you,' I explained.

'Another do-gooder,' sneered Mrs Wimble. I didn't know what to say. 'Well, as you've come uninvited, I suggest you do some good and put the kettle on,' she told me.

Once I'd done what passed for washing-up in this house I was able to present Mrs Wimble with a cup of tea – the milk of which had come direct from her own troublesome nanny goat.

'Not having a brew?' she enquired as she took a sip, her piercing grey eyes fixed on me.

'I had one before I left, thank you,' I excused.

'What did you say your name was?'

'Sarah Hill, the new health visitor.'

'Health visitor indeed. Busybody more like it,' she barked. 'Hmm. Did you say that senile Dr Drake sent you?'

'He did.'

'Was he on this plane or a higher one when he saw fit to poke his beaky nose into my business?' I smiled to myself but I didn't say anything. 'There is something in that meditating lark, I suppose,' continued Mrs Wimble through loud slurps of tea. 'Though I prefer to look to Mother Nature for my remedies.'

'Are you a herbalist?' I enquired.

'Do you take me for a broomstick rider?' Mrs Wimble snapped. 'My late husband and I were both botanists.'

'Really? I loved Botany at school,' I replied enthusiastically.

'Did you indeed?' she cackled. 'All right, Nurse. I'll let you give me the once-over if you can tell me what tree is used to make aspirin.'

I thought back to my tutorials and the piles of open medical books in the reading room of Hackney Nurses' Home and flipped the pages through in my mind's eye until I saw the right one as if it was there in front of me.

'I seem to recall the acetyl ester of salicylic acid was originally isolated from the bark of a tree,' I answered.

The left side of Mrs Wimble's mouth turned up in a lopsided half-smile. 'Ah, but which tree?'

I pictured the drive through her woods trying to recall the texture of the barks. 'The willow tree,' I ventured timidly.

Mrs Wimble didn't tell me if I'd answered her questions correctly. Instead the old lady changed the subject.

'Did you meet Gray, my gander?' she enquired, putting her tea on a side table with a collection of knitting needles. I nodded. 'He saw off that ditsy blonde district nurse last week,' she crowed.

'Nurse Bates?' I enquired.

'Friend of yours?'

'I haven't met her yet. This is my second week in Totley.'

'Don't bother. A girl like that is more interested in polishing nails than trimming them. Wouldn't let her over the threshold let alone let her get her scalpel near my feet.'

I wondered if I'd answered her botany question correctly and decided to try my luck. 'Would you like me to take a look at your feet, Mrs Wimble?'

'If you must,' she replied huffily.

I pulled off her muddy Wellington boots and holey socks. Her feet were dry and sore, her toenails yellow and curling over the edges of her toes. Thick blue veins ran up her legs. She turned her gaze to the window and grumbled before closing her eyes; she couldn't be bothered with me anymore.

I fetched my medical bag and a bowl of warm soapy water. She slept or pretended to nap as I wordlessly bathed her toes, soles, heels and ankles and then trimmed her toenails the best I could. Finally, I rubbed some ointment into her legs and feet and left them elevated on a footstool to dry before I slipped away. My time here had expired for the day, but I would be back. Mrs Wimble had worked her spell on me – I wanted to know more about this intriguing old lady. Somehow, I don't know how, I'd momentarily broken through the impenetrable barrier she'd built around Peasblossom and her solitary life. There wasn't much she'd let me do, but I was determined to do what I could.

# 5

Tuesday afternoon I was back in my broom cupboard before Totley baby clinic. Thanks to Flo I'd opened up with a new set of keys and Mrs Martha Bunyard was none the wiser.

Mrs King appeared. 'Hello, I popped in to see how you are, Miss Hill.'

'They haven't brought anyone through to see me yet.'

'Oh, I see. What are you going to do?'

I noticed one intrepid mum with beautifully waved long auburn hair, who wore a flowing maxi maternity dress in a striped pattern of burnt orange and toffee with a pair of smartly turned-out little girls clutching each of her hands, make her way up to Mrs Martha Bunyard's coven.

'I'd like to see the health visitor please,' she requested politely but firmly.

'You don't really want to pester the new health visitor before she knows what's what. She's terribly busy. Tell me, what's niggling you?'

I was almost on the verge of saying quite rudely that it was no trouble at all and I'd like to be a hundred times busier when Mrs King stepped in with cheerful calm and said to the pregnant mum, 'Ah, Mrs Bourne. This is Miss Hill, your new health visitor – aren't you lucky?' before slipping away again.

'Follow me, Mrs Bourne,' I said calmly but I felt as green as grass. 'Let's find a quiet corner to talk in.'

Mrs Bourne sighed with relief. I turned round the table I'd spotted the day before and put chairs on either side and found a few toys for her children to play with from the toy box to allow us a few minutes of uninterrupted conversation.

After chatting about potty training for about 15 minutes the elegant Mrs Bourne left the clinic with a mutually agreed approach. I'd suggested we catch up in two weeks to see how things were going. Mrs Bourne already had a really good idea of what to do and needed only a few more suggestions and reassurance she was on the right track. It made my blood boil to think that mothers had been turned away from getting a service they had a right to by busybody ladies of the parish. What if they'd had a serious problem, what if it was a matter of life and death? With no medical background who were they to decide who got a service and who didn't? Never mind waiting, I threw caution to the wind and decided with youthful vigour that it was going to be my way or the highway.

Having seen my first client of the afternoon I felt emboldened that she was not going to be the last and returned to Mrs Martha Bunyard and her tea party. I heard her friend Mrs Doris Bowyer muttering, 'Who does think she is? She's just a slip of a girl. I've been lending a helping hand at this clinic for the last 20 years. If it's good enough ...' her voiced trailed away as the third volunteer, Miss Elena Moon, shushed her as they saw me approaching.

'Ladies, I wanted to say thank you so much for giving up your time to help at clinic today and for showing me the ropes last week.' Miss Moon muttered 'You're welcome' but the rest remained tight-lipped. 'Mrs Bunyard,' I continued, locking eyes with this woman who must have only been in her late fifties but to me seemed like Methuselah. 'I think you would be the perfect person to greet and welcome the mothers when they arrive and locate their records for them to give to me.'

'What, trust mothers with their own records?' she said in horror.

'Yes, they can keep hold of them and give in their card when they get their baby weighed, or to me when we do checks and then return it to you before they leave,' I told her.

'Well, I never ...'

'You must know practically every mother and baby in the village,' I suggested.

'I certainly do,' confirmed Mrs Martha Bunyard.

'You will be the face of Totley Clinic – the first point of contact. I would like every mother who comes through these doors to get a warm welcome.'

'Well, I'm sure I can rise to the task, Nurse,' she snapped.

'Perfect,' I enthused. 'Please do ask every mother if they would like to see me. Clinic is much more than getting a baby weighed, don't you think?'

I knew she didn't think that in the slightest but, who knows, in time maybe even Methuselah would come round. I was going to keep a careful eye on Mrs Martha Bunyard and her friends to see how they spoke to the mothers. It was our clients who were the most important people at clinic, not the health visitor and not the ladies who volunteered.

'Mrs Bowyer,' I began, 'Perhaps you could run a little refreshment station for me,' I asked. 'I'm sure you must have lots of catering experience. Keeping our hard-working volunteers, mothers and their little ones hydrated is vital, don't you think?'

'Certainly, Nurse. I'll ask Mrs Farthing if I can use the kitchen.'

'What a good suggestion, thank you.'

And she too scuttled off to take up her new role with a few mutterings and sly glances in my direction.

'Now, Miss Moon, would you mind setting up a play area for me, to help keep the toddlers amused?'

'I will, Nurse,' she replied gently. 'I know exactly where the toy box and the play mats are. I often help my niece at Mums and Toddlers on a Wednesday.'

'Thank you,' I said, beaming. 'I'd like the mothers to have the opportunity to sit down for a rest and a chat with each other as much as anything – it is after all *their* baby clinic. And please do encourage the mums to come and talk to me about anything. Nothing is too much trouble. I won't be in the consulting room from now on – I'll be at my table over there, so any parent can see me if they want to,' I told them.

Ten minutes later the ladies of the parish were all busy with their new roles. I noticed the timid little lady who was employed to sell the tins of baby milk doing a steady trade with barely a word spoken. Now, then, how to tackle the volunteers who weighed the babies? With my usual gusto I charged over to wrestle with my next problem.

'Hello, I'm Sarah Hill. Mrs Kettel, isn't it? How's the weighing going today?'

'Very well, thank you, Nurse. I've weighed half a dozen babies already.'

'That's great. I wanted to ask your opinion on something.'

'Go ahead, Nurse. I've been weighing babies at this clinic for the last eight years. I'm a dabster at it,' said Mrs Kettel proudly.

'Goodness me, what a long time. Do you think the clothes on the baby enable you to note down the most accurate weight?'

'It depends, Nurse. In the winter the woollens certainly weigh more,' said Mrs Kettel thoughtfully. 'Not to mention when they do their business in their nappies.'

'Yes, I imagine that makes quite a difference,' I said.

'I should cocoa,' said Mrs Kettel with a chuckle.

'What do you think we can do to get the most accurate weight?' I asked.

'Not much you can do, Nurse, except weigh them burr,' Mrs Kettel said warily.

'Burr?' I enquired.

'Starkers, Nurse. In the all-together,' mocked Mrs Kettel.

'Ah, well, we understand each other perfectly then,' I replied. 'Please, set up three or four changing tables with a few of those plastic bowls for the babies' clothes to go in when they're burr,' I suggested with a glint in my eye, pointing to the unused equipment.

'Are you taking the mickey, Nurse?' asked Mrs Kettel with raised eyebrows.

'How else can we ensure we get the most accurate weight?'

'But what if they widdle or worse in the scales?' she enquired.

'It's not the end of the world if they do. I'm sure you've got plenty of experience with that sort of thing. It's not something that would put you off your stride, is it?'

'Oh, no,' said Mrs Kettel. 'I've seen it all, Nurse.'

'Perfect. Keep some cleaning things near to hand so you can clean up easily. We wouldn't want the mothers to be embarrassed, would we?'

'Oh no. Most natural thing in the world, Nurse. You leave it to us,' she assured me.

'Excellent, thank you.'

I was determined to say hello to every parent who came to clinic at the very least. When I wasn't chatting to a mother I was on my feet to greet them as they came past Mrs Martha Bunyard and co. But to my surprise the ladies seemed to have taken to their new roles. If appearances were anything to go by then they were having a jolly time greeting mothers, peeking at the babies and getting a little bit of village gossip.

'How's it going?' I breezily asked Mrs Martha Bunyard.

'Very well, Nurse,' answered Miss Elena Moon before she could get a word in. 'We think it's much better this way, don't we, Doris?'

'Oh, yes,' added Mrs Doris Bowyer. 'Helps the shy ones come out of themselves a bit. Sometimes you could barely get a hello out of some of the girls and now they're right jawsy.'

'Yes, I don't know why we didn't do it like this before,' finished Miss Moon.

Mrs Martha Bunyard scowled at her friends' new-found enthusiasm.

'That's very good.' I grinned. 'So, let's check. You greet them, especially taking a bit of time with newcomers to explain they can come and get the baby weighed and talk to me about anything.'

'Yes, yes, yes, Nurse. We've been sending you over a steady stream, haven't we?' barked Mrs Martha Bunyard.

'Yes. Very well organised,' I praised. 'And you are recording all the names in the book as they arrive, giving out the clinic cards and adding in any missing information like date of birth or their address?'

'All in hand, Nurse. You leave it to us,' Mrs Martha Bunyard said firmly.

'Excellent, thank you,' I acknowledged before returning to see how the new system for weighing was progressing.

'It really is much better like this, Martha,' I heard Miss Moon whisper. 'I don't know why we didn't do it like this years ago.'

By Friday morning I'd completed my second week in Totley and lived to tell the tale. In the last 10 days I'd done two baby clinics, 10 primary visits, four follow-up visits, one elderly referral, three call-outs, 15 hearing tests, one school visit complete with extracting a child's head from the school railings and assisted in what I hoped would be my last ever labour. Hermione had told me they were breaking me in gently. It was with great enthusiasm that I now knocked on the peeling red front door of a crumbling cottage to make the primary visit to Mrs Susan Bunyard, whose baby I'd helped deliver not two weeks before. The house stood in the middle of a row of 10 workers' houses opposite the brewery. When the door opened I felt a wave of disappointment when the crabby clinic volunteer Mrs Martha Bunyard, the dreaded mother-in-law no doubt, opened the front door.

'She's using the outdoor convenience, Nurse,' she told me. 'Come through. My daughter and my husband's elder sister have come to have a hold of baby Sharon. I ask you, what sort of name is Sharon? First-born girls in the Bunyard family have always been called Constance, isn't that right?'

The visitors nodded in agreement – I later discovered they were both called Constance. The in-laws were seated on a squat battered brown sofa facing the small open fireplace in front of which was a zinc bathtub. The room was absolutely stifling with a roaring fire lit to heat up the bathwater for when Alan Bunyard returned after a day's graft at the brewery. Baby Sharon looked helpless in the enormous lap of her great-aunt Constance, the poor child making a low continual whimpering noise that they all ignored. I could see through to a small kitchen with an old sink, a single cupboard and an ancient stove. There was no preparation space except for a minuscule flap-down storage unit and a rickety wooden table pushed up against the kitchen wall.

The back door opened and in walked Susan Bunyard. She went directly to the kitchen sink; the plumbing loudly whined into life as she turned on the single tap and washed her hands in a thundering, spluttering stream of cold water with a bar of Camay soap and splashed her face. Hearing her baby's cries she marched into the cramped front room with a face like thunder and snatched back her child as tea cups were being passed over the infant's head. Baby Sharon, clearly relieved to be returned to her mother, who had after all only popped to the outside lavatory, instantly stopped crying and buried her face in her mum's neck. Mrs Bunyard noticed me standing uncomfortably in the corner.

'Oh my, I didn't see you there, Nurse. Nice to see you again,' she greeted me warmly.

'The baby is a right moaning Minnie,' Great-aunt Constance informed her loudly. 'You're spoiling her. She's full of windgines. If I've told you once I've told you a thousand times already, girl. If they are cranky, you take a red-hot poker from the fire and put it in a bottle full of water. Then they drink the cinder water, and throw up all the nasty stuff. Cleans them right out; I've done it with all mine, never did them any harm,' she informed the company with all the overbearing confidence of the depressingly ignorant.

'Well, she's not having a bottle yet, she's on the breast,' Susan Bunyard diplomatically informed this interfering old biddy.

'That's another thing, Nurse,' chipped in Mrs Martha Bunyard. 'I've told her to put the baby on the National Dried, but she won't have it. She's crying because you're not feeding her right, girl. She needs feeding up; you need to put her on the bottle before she wastes away. All my babies were right whackers.'

Oh, the horror of unwanted baby advice, I thought, digging my fingernails into the palm of my hand. I looked at Mrs Bunyard; there was no doubt in my mind she knew this was all total rubbish. The new mother's eyes were narrowing, her cheeks getting pinker and pinker by the second. I didn't know if she was going to scream or cry. She raised her eyes to the ceiling with a pleading look in my direction.

'I need to check your tummy, Mrs Bunyard,' I said clearly, picking up the desperate hint. 'Is the bedroom upstairs?'

'Follow me, Nurse,' she told me, keeping the baby firmly clutched to her chest as she opened a small wooden door off the kitchen that led up a narrow twisted staircase to the two tiny rooms above.

'You do that, Nurse,' said Mrs Martha Bunyard, giving me her unnecessary assurance. 'And take a look at baby Sharon's belly button. I don't trust that Nurse Higgins. I don't believe she trained in a proper English hospital. She's cut the cord all wrong and given the baby a sticky-out belly button; it looks black as your hat too.'

Don't say anything, Sarah, just get upstairs, I told myself. My chest was tight, I was burning to tell these women how foolish and harmful their pestering was. Not now, not now, I had to repeat to myself.

'You can't trust 'em,' agreed her daughter, Connie, returning to their disparagement of the lovely midwife. 'I swear it's some voodoo. She did it to all four of mine but I fixed it. Got a penny off one of them gypsies and bound it round the baba till it went back in again,' she said proudly.

Susan Bunyard had already fled up the dilapidated staircase like lightning, eager to get away. As we closed the door on the three Bunyard matriarchs slurping their tea I heard Great-aunt Constance give the most dim-witted piece of baby advice I'd heard yet.

'That baby probably has thrush. I've told her if you wipe their wet-cloth nappy on their tongue it clears up straight away. But she doesn't take heed. She's not a Kentish girl. She's from Essex, so what do you expect? I don't know what your Alan was thinking, Martha.'

I firmly shut the door on them. It would not be the last time I had to watch mothers taunted with ill-conceived baby advice that was sometimes well meant but other times was nasty, cruel and harmful.

Mrs Bunyard was on the bed feeding her lovely baby, propped up by pillows to shield her back from the uncomfortable brass bars of the headboard. Her wide square-necked peasant shirt was just the job for nursing. She'd pulled her long sandy-coloured hair into a messy bun and looked different to how she was only moments before. Relaxed and contented now she was alone with her baby, I could see what a strong bond they had already: it was beautiful.

'You don't mind, do you?' she asked.

'Not at all. You look like you're doing a splendid job. How was last week?'

'It was all right when it was just me and Sharon. But it's hell when his lot are traipsing in and out of the place. Wanting cups of tea and giving me filthy looks if I offer them shop-bought cake. Where would I get the time to make bloody cake for the hordes that have been through here?' she told me indignantly.

'Could Mr Bunyard help keep some of the visitors at bay?'

'He's as much use as a wet tea towel, Nurse. He likes to play the doting daddy but it's like having another kid to look after. He made a big show of changing Sharon's nappy last night and stuck a pin in her!' she told me, her eyes filled with exasperation.

'But he does want to help?' I asked tentatively.

'What would help me out is a proper bathroom with an indoor toilet, hot and cold water, and a proper plumbed-in bath for Lord's sake,' she cried. 'I'm not used to living like this – it's like something out of a BBC olde-worlde drama. My parents' house has all mod cons, thank you very much. My mother had a properly fitted kitchen – she never had to try and turn out a dinner on a clapped-out stove. He says he'll get onto the brewery about updating the cottages but they've been promising to modernise since after the war apparently. I've said the men and him need to get organised, demand proper housing, but they couldn't organise …' her voice trailed away as she paused to change the baby's nappy, spreading out the terry towelling on the bed and then washing her hands in a ceramic bowl and jug of water on a wash stand.

'It's like I'm in a bloody episode of *Upstairs, Downstairs*,' she said with a grim laugh. 'Only you imagine you'll be one of ladies in fancy dresses, not living like a charwoman.'

I nipped down to the kitchen to fetch her a glass of water. When I returned, baby Sharon was feeding steadily on the other side.

'I've brought you some cake,' I said as I put a tray on the bedside table with a jug of water and a big slice of Victoria sponge cake on it.

'Thank you, Nurse. You shouldn't have,' she said, drinking down her water in almost one go.

'Yes, I should. You need to rest and get plenty to eat and drink if you're going to keep on doing such a fabulous job feeding little Sharon.'

'You don't think she's underweight? Honestly she doesn't cry that much.'

As the baby came off the breast all satisfied and sleepy I had a quick hold, while Mrs Bunyard ate her cake. I took the opportunity to give her a full MOT, discreetly checking everything was as it should be – she was perfect.

'She seems just right to me.'

'I know what his lot think, that I'm no good. That I should give the baby to them. Well, no one is taking this baby off me; I'd die first than let them take her away. They won't take her away, will they, Nurse?'

'No one is going to take your baby away – please don't worry about that.'

'They try and make out that she never stops crying but it's not true. I think she cries sometimes because she wants her mum, or because everything is a bit new and she wants a bit of comfort – I know how she feels.'

'That sounds right to me. You know your baby best, Mrs Bunyard. You really are doing a splendid job.'

Susan Bunyard grinned and took the baby to a large wicker crib and popped her daughter down for a nap.

'She's kept me up a lot in the night, though. Are you sure she's getting enough milk?'

'Are you getting lots of wet and dirty nappies?' I asked.

'There's an endless stream,' she laughed. 'Her poo's all yellow, though.'

'Yes, that's how it should be. How she's sleeping during the day?'

'She's an angel in the day. When will you come back, Nurse?'

'End of next week if it suits you?'

'Yes, that would be great. And hopefully the Wicked Witch of the West won't be here,' she whispered.

'Do you want to lie down flat and I'll take a look at your tummy?' I asked her.

As I pressed down on her belly she gazed up at the cracks in the low ceiling above the marital bed and said in a whisper almost more to herself than to me, 'I'd never change having Sharon. But I'm not sure if I did the right thing marrying Aly.'

'It's normal to feel worried and a bit overwhelmed at times,' I tried to reassure her.

There was a long pause. 'Nurse, if I tell you something, will you keep it a secret?' she asked.

'Absolutely,' I replied.

She opened her mouth but no words came out. I waited.

'It's about Aly, he doesn't …' But before she could finish telling me the door to the narrow staircase opened and Alan Bunyard called up.

'I took an early lunch break. I couldn't wait to see my girls,' he cried as he bound up the rickety stairs.

Mrs Bunyard instantly brightened and rushed to her makeshift dressing table to brush her hair back into place.

'Don't mind me, Nurse. I'm being silly,' she told me as her husband reached the top but she didn't look me in the eye again.

Mr Bunyard rushed in and picked up the slumbering baby without a thought of how long she may have been sleeping – not long at all as it happened. I packed up my things; the visit was now over. We all have secrets, that's normal, and Mrs Bunyard wasn't under any obligation to tell her secret but since I first laid eyes on this young woman, who was only 19, I couldn't help but notice she didn't have the bloom of a new bride and mother. She was troubled; something was not what it seemed. 'I can't put my finger on it,' I mused as I left the Bunyard household.

*6*

After my run-in with the baby-clinic volunteers I didn't show my face at the Totley Mums and Toddlers group until the end of September. I didn't want to give the impression that I was coming in and taking over everything and thought I knew it all – because most of the time it felt like I knew barely anything at all. Hospital life had been simpler, the lines distinct. I had been a nurse with a very clear purpose in a strict hierarchy. Yes, I might have found myself in hot water with Sister or Matron on occasion, but here, well, it was like trying to get your head round all the intricacies of a long-running show like *The Archers* after listening for only a week or two; you didn't know who was who and you felt like you were constantly stumbling across intrigues and old family feuds. Nothing was clear-cut anymore – community practice in an area like Totley was a constant overlapping of never-ending stories and problems and history that I couldn't possibly ever know. Eight hundred families and up – how was I ever to get them all straight in my head? Added to which I'd not been able to see Mrs Susan Bunyard and baby Sharon. Every time I went she was out. I was concerned I'd done something wrong and she was avoiding me.

It had reached a point where if I didn't pop into Mums and Toddlers rather than looking interfering it might appear that I couldn't care less, and didn't think it worth my time. I determined I would try not to get in the way or hinder the natural chat that occurs between mothers with children the same age. I would try and show them I was there should they ever want me – 'Why would they want you?' piped up the unhelpful voice in my head. On the way to the Village Hall I passed the baker's and was surprised to see Hermione Drummond through the window, chatting animatedly to two men. I caught her eye and she waved me in enthusiastically, her strings of glass beads jostling as her arms moved back and forth excitedly.

'Miss Hill, have you tried a Totley freshly baked bun with a sausage from Treetops Farm?' she enquired the second I stepped over the threshold. 'They are devilishly scrumptious,' she informed me, taking a big bite. The baker behind the counter in his white apron looked thrilled as he watched Hermione eat with rapture.

'I haven't had one yet,' I replied.

'One more please, Bob,' Hermione called to the baker, who jumped to her command. 'I don't want you thinking I normally slope off, Miss Hill, but I've a case conference at 11 o'clock and it's likely to go on for hours and I stupidly skipped breakfast.' Her eyes turned back to the men. 'So, I thought I'd have an illicit banger butty,' she hooted, her voice chiming like a cathedral bell. 'And who should I find truanting but a schoolmaster and a Man of the Cloth,' she teased, giving the older of the two men a pat on the shoulder.

'Miss Hill, have you met Mr Hopkins, the headmaster at St Agatha's, and the Reverend Nicholas Shepherd, our dashing new vicar?'

'We haven't,' responded the older man. 'Dylan Hopkins. Pleasure to meet our new school nurse. I think you spoke to my deputy when you popped into the school, Miss Hill,' he said, grinning and firmly shaking my hand. 'Miss Drummond is right, I am a fugitive from playground duty but Father Nick and I are discussing the school trip to Canterbury Cathedral this Saturday. We are trying to form a plan of action for volunteers. Miss Drummond, I believe you have already thrown your hat into the ring?'

Hermione sucked on a buttery finger. 'Oh, yes, count me in, for better or for worse.' Her brown eyes were brilliant with mischief as she held me in her gaze and suggested, 'And I'm sure Miss Hill would only be too happy to help?', taking another mouthful of her sandwich.

I gulped. Suddenly Mr Hopkins and the Reverend Shepherd seemed to be closing in on me in the confines of the village bakery. I hadn't really noticed the rector properly until now, all eyes being on Hermione. The preacher had dark wavy hair, curling in thick glossy ringlets over his collar; surely his hair was a bit too long for a Man of the Cloth? And despite the dog collar he was rather cool in a white and brown checked sports jacket teamed with fawn slacks. He had huge dark eyes and eyelashes so long they looked fake.

'That would help get us out of a huge hole if you could face the pilgrimage,' added Mr Hopkins. 'Wouldn't it, Reverend Shepherd?'

'Right on,' replied the cool country parson, his eyes still fixed on me. I tried not to squirm under the gaze of this tower of a man.

'I'd be happy to help,' I replied over-brightly.

'Excellent,' Mr Hopkins said, clapping his hands together. 'I'll leave Miss Drummond to fill you in on the details. Father Nick and I have to get back for morning assembly.'

They stepped out of the cramped bakery, their illicit baked goods in hand. The Reverend turned back to look at me from the narrow doorway; he blocked the light and the sunlight formed a ring round his black mop of hair.

'See you Saturday,' he crooned.

Then they left. I was glad. Hermione passed me my sausage sandwich.

'Hasn't he got heavenly eyelashes?' said Hermione smoothly.

'The Headmaster?' I spluttered.

Hermione sighed. 'No. Mr Hopkins isn't the overpowering good-looking type. More of a slow burn.'

I didn't reply but nibbled my sandwich. Oh, it was delicious. Say what you like about Joe Rudcliff, he obviously produced good porkers. My trip to the bakery must have been divine intervention as I remembered if there is one thing I've learnt about mums' groups, it is that delectable cake and a decent cup of coffee are the cornerstone of a successful morning meeting. I immediately invested in a large carrot cake. Next time I'd go one better and bake it myself with a recipe for apple cake from the Friends of the Earth cookbook, my newlywed friend Fiona Flemming had sent me as a moving-in present. I could use the honey from Clem's bees, I mused, momentarily distracted by thoughts of bucolic country living, the humming of bees and dishy clergymen.

Mums and toddlers was already under way when I arrived with my baked goods. A young woman about my age, wearing an emerald green shirt tucked into the same colour flared trousers with a thin white belt round her waist, and a green and white striped headscarf covering thick dark blonde curls, sat cross-legged in a circle with the other mums and children, leading the singing.

One, two, three, four, five,
Once I caught a fish alive,
Six, seven, eight, nine, ten,
Then I let it go again.

About half the mothers joined in, mainly the ones with a single toddler in their laps. The other half were in little huddles, gossiping, some with children hanging off their arms, whining for attention, while other toddlers were taking the opportunity to get into cupboards, hide under tables, squabble over toys or have a sulk in a corner.

> Why did you let it go?
> Because it bit my finger so.
> Which finger did it bite?
> This little finger on the right.

The group leader finished, with the few mums who remained in the circle snapping and kissing the fingers of their offspring and tickling them as they lay giggling and kicking in their laps.

'Please help yourself to squash and biscuits,' announced the group leader as she finished, her eyes already roving the room. There was no child in her lap. I went forward with my carrot cake and tried to put aside my immediate horror that they were serving the children squash. They'll be whizzing around like spinning tops in no time, I thought.

I introduced myself. 'Hello, I'm Sarah Hill, the new health visitor.'

'Oh, we know who you are, Nurse,' called one of the mums in the circle as she bounced a bonny baby on her knee. Her little girl was about a year old with mustard-coloured corduroy dungarees and a multi-coloured star T-shirt, and I could make out a sizeable bump under her the mum's loose denim shirt.

I smiled. The mums exchanged not unfriendly glances. 'I wanted to drop off a cake for the group,' I explained, thrusting forward my goodwill offering.

'Ooh, what is it?' asked the expectant mum, putting her toddling little one down to explore.

'It's a carrot cake,' I explained.

'Not had that before but we'll give it a whirl. I am eating for two after all,' she remarked cheerily, taking the carrot cake off my hands. 'Miss Elena, would you do the honours please?' she asked an older lady, who I recognised as one of my kinder helpers at the baby clinic.

'With pleasure,' answered Miss Elena Moon, fresh from the kitchen carrying a tray of cups, which she handed out with care to the mums.

I smiled at the group leader but she was still distracted. 'Aunty Elena, have you seen Dean?' she asked.

'No, dear, I haven't,' answered Miss Moon. 'He did pop into the kitchen a little while ago for a biscuit but I haven't seen him since.'

'Would you like me to help look for him?' I asked.

'Please. I'm probably just panicking. But he won't sit still and join in with the singing. He takes himself off,' she explained, her eyes still anxiously scanning the room.

'What does he look like?'

'Oh, sorry. I'm Yvonne. Yvonne Underdown. His name's Dean. He's three. Curly light brown hair and he's wearing blue jeans and a red T-shirt.'

Our somewhat half-hearted small search party spread out peeking under tables and rifling through cupboards but there was no sign of him.

'I hope he hasn't wandered out onto the road,' said Mrs Underdown, her voice high and breathless.

'She's always getting herself in a lather,' hissed the pregnant mum to a friend, a bit too loudly to be classed as a whisper.

'I'll check the kitchen again,' I suggested.

I stood and surveyed the unloved kitchen. All outdated cupboards almost off their hinges and piles of plastic cups and plates in the huge stainless steel skin waiting to be washed. There was definitely a banging noise coming from somewhere. I opened the lower cupboards one by one until I found a boy in blue jeans and a red T-shirt, but I couldn't be sure of the colour of his hair as he had a saucepan stuck firmly over the top of his head.

'Found him, Mrs Underdown,' I called as I gently lifted the boy out of the cupboard.

Mrs Underdown rushed in and let out a huge sigh of relief quickly followed by shouting. 'Dean, you tiresome child! You know you're not to wander off and now look at you. You wait till your father gets home, you little horror.'

'Oh dear, oh dear,' gasped Miss Moon. 'What shall we do? We'll have to take him to hospital and get the doctor to saw it off.'

Dean let out a wail and started hitting the pan with his fists.

'No need for that,' I said calmly. 'Can you find me some cooking oil please, Miss Moon.' The dutiful great-aunt raided every kitchen cupboard until she returned with an old bottle of vegetable cooking oil in her trembling hand. I addressed the saucepan head. 'Hello, Dean. I'm a nurse. I want you to hold still while I put some oil into the saucepan to get your head free. It won't hurt but it will feel a bit sticky,' I told him.

And a minute or two later a curly-haired, rather oily little boy's face appeared. His nose was a bit squashed but he looked perfectly fine. I rubbed his head with a tea towel.

'Look at the state of you,' cried Mrs Underdown as she hugged him to her chest, getting oil all over her clothes. 'Home now. You're going straight in the bath.'

'Not my fault. Soldier told me to,' he whined as his mother tucked him under her arm and strode out of the kitchen.

'Stop making up silly stories,' she scolded him. As she reached the doorway she turned and tried to compose herself. 'I'm sorry, Nurse. It's not usually like this.'

'Happy to help,' I replied, washing my hands in the sink.

'Thank you,' said Mrs Underdown as she turned on her heel and stormed off, her Aunty Elena following behind her in a complete tizzy.

'That boy's a bit soft,' said the pregnant mum who'd been eager to try my carrot cake. 'No wonder Yvonne's flustered. She's got a boy talking to himself in corners like a loony and a husband that's not far off his dotage.'

I turned to her and said. 'I'm sorry I didn't catch your name?'

'Oh, yes. I'm Jackie Bowyer and that one's Stacy,' she indicated to her infant. 'We're neighbours sort of. My husband, Trev, keeps the garage opposite your digs. We live over the shop so to speak.'

'Pleased to meet you, Mrs Bowyer. When's the baby due?'

She now took a big bite of the carrot cake. 'November. Gosh, this is tasty, Nurse. Much nicer than Miss Elena's dry old fruit cake,' she said, giggling. 'Here, girls, try a piece,' she called to the other mums handing the plates around as a group of mothers descended upon us, feeding themselves with one hand and crumbling bits of cake and popping it into the eager mouths of their tots.

'Do you serve cake at the baby clinic too?' asked Mrs Bowyer with a wry smile as she scooped up her baby, who was rooting through the contents of her large fuchsia shoulder bag and chewing the edge of a packet of Benson & Hedges. 'Oi, Stacy, you'll get them all soggy,' chided her mother, wiping the drool-covered pack on her jeans before she pocketed them. I really hoped she wasn't smoking during her pregnancy.

The door opened and in lumbered Mrs Bourne with little girls in tow.

'Sorry we're late. Have we missed the singing again?' she asked wearily.

'Don't worry, you've made it for the most important bit. The nurse brought some cake,' answered Mrs Bowyer.

'That's music to my ears. Run off and play, you two,' she told her children, planting glittering lipstick-smeared kisses on their foreheads before flopping down into a chair. 'Nice to see you again, Nurse,' she said, multi-tasking as she massaged her own pregnant belly with one hand and gobbled some cake with the other. 'You've been the talk of the village,' she told me through a mouthful of crumbs.

'Have I?' I asked, trying to sound amused but feeling suddenly anxious.

'I should cocoa,' said Mrs Bowyer, laughing. 'Trev's mum kept him chatting at the garage till past supper time, telling him all the juicy details after you trounced old Mother Bunyard.'

'How old is baby Stacy?' I asked, trying to change the subject.

'Are you kidding me?' continued Mrs Bowyer, undeterred. 'My mother-in-law is Doris Bowyer. Her and Miss Loopy Loo Elena have been under the thumb of Martha Bunyard for years, though in truth Doris is no better than she ought to be. And then you come along, same age as all of us, your first month in the village and it's a bloody revolution.'

'That's a huge exaggeration,' I said, trying to laugh it off.

'Don't be modest, Nurse. I can tell you're not going to be snooty like some of them. I think you should stick to your guns – don't let them old biddies rule the roost.'

'She's quite right, Nurse,' said Mrs Bourne softly. 'They needed taking down a peg or two. Would it be greedy to have a tiny bit more cake?'

'With pleasure,' I said, giving her another slice. 'I could make some apple cake another time.'

'You can come again,' said Mrs Bowyer, winking. She looked at her watch, 'Gosh, it's nearly 12. Better get back to do the lunch or Trev the Rev will be giving me my marching orders,' she said with a chuckle, retrieving Stacy from the corner where she'd dragged her mother's handbag and emptied out lipstick, face powder, loose change and tampons. Mrs Bowyer shook her head and started putting her paraphernalia back in the bag. 'Oh no! My pill's gone. Stacy, what have you done?' she cried, opening up her child's mouth with a finger. 'Nurse, Nurse. I think she's gobbled my pill.'

'Contraceptive pill?'

'Yes. What'll happen to her?'

'She should be fine. But let's ask the doctor to check her out. He'll probably tell you to keep a close eye on her for 24 hours.'

She nodded. 'You must think we're a right load of Calamity Janes,' she said without her usual giggle, her forehead furrowed.

'Not in the least,' I said. 'Come over to clinic with me now and we'll call the doctor and get him to see Stacy straight away.'

'Thanks, Nurse. Whatever they say, I like you,' Mrs Bowyer assured me.

'You're not still taking your contraceptive pill are you, Mrs Bowyer?'

'No, I haven't got round to chucking 'em away from before we started trying for Stacy,' she laughed. 'Mind I wish I had been taking them, though now this one is on the way, it'll be very welcome.'

'You didn't plan on having another baby so soon?'

'You'd of thought I'd have worked out after having my older two, Jenny and Neil, a year apart that breastfeeding doesn't stop you getting pregnant.'

'No, you can definitely get pregnant while breastfeeding.'

'Will you tell that slimey Dr Botten that for me.'

'Why, did he tell you that you couldn't get pregnant while breastfeeding?'

'He did, Nurse. Can we see Dr Drake? I know he's 103 but he's a nice old boy.'

I smiled and tried to supress my urges to charge in and tear Dr Botten off a strip.

# 7

Sitting in the saloon bar with a book was not how I was used to spending my Friday evenings. Here I was, now way past the legal age for alcoholic consumption on my tod, waiting for my colleagues to celebrate my first month in Totley with a ginger beer, reading one of the many books on the benefits of Transcendental Meditation Dr Drake had given me. The mighty tome I was flicking through – Harold Bloomfield's latest book *TM: Discovering Inner Energy and Overcoming Stress* – the aged GP had informed me was hot off the press. So far, it was not proving to be an easy read. I skimmed through and decided rather than reading it right now, I'd do that activity both procrastinators and methodical people alike love to do: make a list.

*Things to do:*
Read TM book
Dig garden and weed
Cut grass
Prune
Plant vegetables

I looked thoughtfully at my list. It all looked like such hard work; I thought people came to the country to relax. A whole weekend off would have been a luxury in nursing, but what would have been on my list then? Trip to Biba, London Zoo, night at the theatre, dinner at Schmitt's? Either way, it would have meant a night out with the girls or a date – no such luck in Totley. The irony I was sitting in a public house with a painting of Oliver Cromwell over the door did not pass me by. I felt saintly, never mind puritanical. It seemed apt that Totley's village pub was called The Good Intent. Was nun-like existence in my mid-twenties an inevitable part of being a village health visitor?

The bar was propped up by farm labourers and men from the brewery drinking from half-barrel glasses. The brewers loyally partook of Totley Beer while the farm labourers favoured the landlord's homemade scrumpy. The roof was low and had dusty black beams, and the tables and chairs looked as if they'd been in use since the time of the Roundheads and the Cavaliers. There wasn't another woman in sight. Sliding down in the high-backed booth I began to wonder if Hermione and Mrs King were playing a joke on me – we'd said six o'clock and it was almost seven. Surely, they wouldn't stand me up, I told myself. With an unfortunate lack of occupation I was considering turning my attention back to the TM book when to my great relief Hermione burst through the doors and sauntered across to the bar. There was an unmistakable parting of the crowds as the men jostled to make room for the dashing Miss Drummond.

'Sarah, my sweet, I hope you haven't been waiting too long,' Hermione greeted me, kissing me on both cheeks now we were off-duty. 'Beatie's just behind me – wouldn't you know it, we both got a call as we were heading off to join you? Still, a ringing phone must be answered, but now we're free as birds. What's your poison?'

'I'm having ginger beer.'

'Evening, Ted,' Hermione greeted the landlord. 'I'll have a small glass of that divine Beaujolais you brought back with you on your last voyage and a ginger beer for Sister Sarah – she's parked her two mules outside,' Hermione informed him, throwing her head back in laughter and giving me a gentle poke in the ribs. She was so full of joie de vivre it was impossible to take offence. 'Oh, and Mrs King will have an apple ale if you've got any left after the last batch exploded. Is your cellar man's eye on the mend?'

'Mended nicely, thank you, Miss Drummond. You ladies sit down and I'll bring it over. Will you be having the soup tonight?'

'Yes, bring us over a large pan with some of Bob's lovely loaves, will you. What other goodies have you smuggled back with you from across the pond?'

'A dollop of bric and some pâté sound about right?'

'Sounds divine, Ted,' Hermione smiled and picked up our drinks and led me back to our booth.

Once Mrs Beatie King was also ensconced in our corner of The Good Intent, Hermione lifted her glass.

'Let's toast Sarah's first month. Long may she reign.'

Mrs King laughed and we clicked glasses. I'd ditched the ginger beer and moved onto the Beaujolais – I felt very sophisticated.

'We hear your arrival has not been without incident,' teased Hermione.

'It has been more eventful than I expected,' I answered and looked at my drink, not sure what they'd make of my antics.

'Don't worry, we never talk shop here,' Mrs King said gently.

'Snugs have great big lugholes,' elaborated Hermione. 'What I'd like to know is what you make of that rather dishy vicar?'

'Mr Shepherd?' enquired Mrs King, only slightly raising an eyebrow.

'We've only said two words to each other, so I don't make anything at all,' I replied.

'Sarah volunteered to come on the school trip to Canterbury Cathedral tomorrow,' continued Hermione, unperturbed. 'The hand of God looked rather thrilled when you offered to come along.'

'You volunteered me,' I reminded her.

'Did I?' asked Hermione, looking like butter wouldn't melt. 'I don't recall. We have to be gentle with the Reverend Shepherd – we are his virgin parish,' she added, keeping the smirk from her lips.

'Is Mr Hopkins going on the trip?' asked Mrs King as she sipped her apple ale.

'He is,' answered Hermione. 'I was going to beg a favour, Beatie. Could you pop in and check Etty has eaten the food I'll leave for her in the morning, you know what's she's like. More chance of her getting through a box of liquor chocolates than eating some nourishing homemade food.'

'Of course. Or why doesn't she come to us?'

'Wouldn't Jack mind?'

'Of course not. They're a jawsy pair once they get going. It'll give me a chance to get some baking done and stock up the freezer.'

'Oh yes, you've got that lovely new deep freezer. I do envy you. The way prices are going up these days it'll pay for itself. At least here we can grow our own if we've a mind to. Imagine all those poor mothers in high-rise flats in the towns and cities trying to feed a family on their meagre housekeeping. I'm all for women working if they want to, but a mother being forced to leave her baby when she doesn't want to for a few extra pounds in her purse is a sad thing indeed.'

'Yes. I'll be interested to hear what Dr Mia Kellmer Pringle has to say about it at the quarterly meeting,' added Mrs King.

'The Director of the National Children's Bureau?' I asked, surprised and impressed.

'Yes, dear,' replied Mrs King. 'The next meeting is towards the end of October. You'll have a chance to meet the wider caring community if you haven't already. It's a good opportunity to exchange news and we always have a speaker.'

'Yes, Miss Presnell really pulled a rabbit out of the hat with getting Mia Kellmer Pringle,' agreed Hermione, draining her glass.

'Have you read *The Needs of Children*?' enquired Mrs King.

'I've heard of it … but I've not actually read it,' I confessed.

'Would you like me to lend you a copy?'

'That's very kind,' I enthused, adding the book to my mental list of improving things to do. 'But it will be a good excuse for me to visit the library and bookshop in Malling.'

'Oh yes, do,' encouraged Hermione. 'The library is closed on Sunday of course, but open the rest of the week and on Tuesdays they host a rather renowned local history group. The bookshop runs a little reading club too – I often like to join in. Though I must admit, I am a devotee of the Collins Crime Club for Agatha Christie alone. We are all on tenterhooks waiting for *Curtain: Poirot's Last Case*.'

'Really, I love Agatha Christie.' I moved Monsieur Poirot to the top of my 'to be read pile' – my professional improvement could wait.

'I knew I liked you the minute I met you,' said Hermione with a titter. 'Why don't we read it together? It'll be a hoot. I bet we'll discover many a copy tucked away during visits. What about you, Beatie?'

'Knitting and baking are more how I spend my few leisure hours,' replied Mrs King. Hermione looked momentarily dispirited. 'But for you I will make an exception. Count me in,' she added, grinning.

We were merrily chomping through the landlord's delicious assortment of breads and cheeses after some very hearty soup when Ernestine Higgins, the midwife, strolled in with a very attractive blonde bombshell. Nurse Higgins was resplendent off-duty, her thick dark curls with that perfect streak of white were now free from the confines of her pillbox hat and fell loosely to her shoulders. She couldn't have picked a more striking contrast to her navy starched uniform as she wafted, in in a white, green and peach print dress with plastic beads wrapped round both her wrists.

'Evening, my sweets,' she called. 'What a fine gathering you make,' she added with a chuckle as she edged her well-built body into the booth.

The girl scowled at me. Her bright-cherry-coloured lips pursed and her eyes narrowed in hostile silence.

'Sit down, sweetness,' Nurse Higgins told her. 'Make yourself comfortable.'

The girl flicked her glossy blonde locks and sharply sat down, crossing her long bare legs and edging down her pale-pink skirt with buttons all down the front. Her left shin had a large plaster over it. She resolutely folded her arms underneath the bust of her tight white T-shirt embroidered with rosy flowers and leaves. She'd have been extremely pretty if her face hadn't been so sour.

'And now our circle is complete. Time to enjoy one of life's lovely moments,' announced Hermione. 'Ernestine, I think you were first off the mark to meet our new arrival, Sarah?'

'Oh yes,' said Nurse Higgins with a chuckle. 'We're already firm friends, aren't we?' I grinned in reply.

'Have you met our district nurse, Miss Bates? She's only been with us a few months but she's already a firm favourite,' explained Hermione.

'Only to some,' huffed the blonde district nurse.

'Well, I think it's time we had another drink. Another apple ale, Beatie?'

'No, thanks. It's almost eight and I said I'd be back to watch *Dad's Army* with Jack and the boys. He'll be back from the fish and chip shop any minute,' said Mrs King, collecting her handbag and wrapping a lovely lilac chiffon scarf around her neck.

'Sounds like bliss,' Hermione told her and I must admit it did.

'Though I don't know if I'll be able to manage anything after all this,' sighed Mrs King, looking at the empty dishes on our table.

'A little bit of what you fancy does you good,' Hermione encouraged. 'Ernestine, give me a hand getting a round in, would you? I think we'll have a bottle of Beaujolais this time. Care to join me, girls?'

I smiled and Miss Bates gave a curt nod of the head.

'A fruit cup for me,' Nurse Higgins said. 'One of us needs to be sober in case there's an emergency and I wouldn't want to be pulled over for drunk driving by my own husband,' she added with a chuckle.

'Is your husband a policeman?'

'He is – he's based in Maidstone but he does cover the village when the occasion calls.'

'Oh, I saw a mum there in one of those nice new police houses,' I replied.

'We used to have one of those,' Ernestine said quietly.

'Come on, Ernestine, those drinks won't get themselves,' insisted Hermione.

Nurse Bates and I remained in an uncomfortable silence. Hermione and Nurse Higgins seemed to be taking an elongated amount of time to get the drinks in. I didn't know whether to try and engage her or ride out her taciturnity. Was it me, or did she seem unaccountably hostile?

'How long have you been a district nurse?' I tried.

'Longer than you've been a health visitor,' she sneered.

I looked at her skin more closely. Underneath the pale make-up her complexion was good. She was only three or four years older than me at a guess. I had hoped we'd be friends.

'You didn't want to live in the village?' I asked. It was meant as a question but it came out like an accusation, to her ear anyway.

'Been listening to yokel tittle-tattle, have we?' she told me off. 'Well, I'm not one to poke my nose in where it's not wanted.'

I was extremely perplexed. Why was she being such a shrew? 'Miss Bates, we seem to have got off on the wrong foot, I'm not sure how, but have I done something to upset you?'

'Upset me? Upset me! What am I, some wet-behind-the-ears student nurse? All I expect is some professional courtesy, is that too much to ask?'

I'd had enough. 'What are you talking about?' I demanded.

'I'm talking about going and treating my patients, acting like I can't do my job, that's what I'm talking about.'

But I still didn't understand. I tried to get some specifics. 'What patient?'

'What patient? What patient!'

'Yes, what patient?'

'Mrs Wimble,' she snarled. 'I went to call her on this afternoon and was told in no uncertain terms that I wasn't required. That the new health visitor had been and seen her already, and that I needn't call again.' She folded her arms tight against her chest and stared resolutely at the wall behind my head.

I let her simmer down for a moment before I asked my last question. 'Did the guard goose nearly have your leg off too?'

Her eyes slid back to me and unblinking held my gaze. 'I had to administer first aid in my Morris Minor,' she told me seriously, flexing her injured left leg for my inspection.

I bit my lip. 'Oh dear.'

'Did Dr Drake send you?' asked Nurse Bates.

'He did. But only because he wanted me to take a gander at the old lady before he called the welfare department. I was a last resort.'

Her eyes bore into me. 'Did he give you that book on that meditation lark?' she asked, tapping on the indigestible hardback on the table. I nodded. 'I don't believe in any of that stuff,' she said tartly. 'Nor in Mrs Wimble's plant voodoo – I think it's,' she paused and said slowly, 'prop-a-gander,' she informed me, staring me out. And then we both started to laugh, banging our hands on the table in a release of pent-up anger, worry and fear.

'Oh, Miss Hill, that bloody goose! Nothing would give me greater pleasure than to serve it up on Christmas Day,' cried Miss Bates as Hermione and Nurse Higgins returned with a much-needed bottle of Beaujolais and one fruit cup.

'I see you two are getting on nicely,' Hermione commented.

'I was telling Sarah how much I'd like to cook Mrs Wimble's goose,' Miss Bates informed her.

Hermione frowned. Then she said most clearly:

If your lips would keep from slips,
Five things observe with care –
Of whom you speak,
To whom you speak,
And how and when and where.

Quite rightly reprimanded we stuck to slightly safer topics of food, books, TV and men.

## 8

Ring, ring. Ring, ring. Ring, ring. The telephone rudely awoke me. For heaven's sake, I thought, it's Saturday morning, this better be a medical emergency. Stumbling out of bed, I crossed the landing, using the walls and door frames for support as the telephone summoned me onwards with its incessant ringing. Everything was still a little blurry. I tripped over a pair of platform white ankle boots and banged my leg on the kitchen table. As I crossly rubbed my smarting shins I eyed the boots suspiciously. 'Those aren't my boots,' I may have said out loud. There was a light snort in response coming from the other side of my sofa. I peeked over the top and saw the comatose figure of District Nurse Laura Bates in the foetal position, using my navy reefer jacket as a makeshift blanket. Laura was slumbering unashamedly with her face turned into the sofa cushions, with one of my old cardigans pulled over her ears to block out the ceaseless trilling telephone. I crossed one hand over the other and used the edge of the sofa as my final aid until I reached the telephone on a side table.

'Hello,' I answered weakly.

'Sarah, I'm on my way to the school now to meet the bus,' Hermione breezed. 'Do you have a first-aid kit you could bring? Only I lent mine to Brown Owl last week and she hasn't returned it yet.'

Oh Lord. It was the school trip to Canterbury. I'd completely forgotten.

'Oh yes, Hermione. I'll bring one, no problem. I was on my way myself,' I lied.

'Perfect. See you in two ticks,' Hermione said brightly before hanging up.

'Laura, wake up. I've got to get going. I'm supposed to be chaperoning St Agatha's school trip to Canterbury right now,' I informed my new friend, tapping her lightly and repeatedly on the back.

'He who would valiant be / 'Gainst all disaster,' sang Laura. 'Will you be going by donkey or car?' she giggled.

'A clapped-out school bus, probably,' I replied.

'They tried to rope me into that last week. Mr Hopkins cornered me in the village shop but there's no way I'm putting up with those snotty officers' wives all day. Bored RAF matriarchs and village tearaways are a toxic mix.'

'They didn't mention anything about RAF wives.'

'Is that dishy new vicar going?' asked Laura, suddenly bright-eyed and upright. I didn't want to commit to thinking Nick Shepherd was dishy, so I just nodded.

'I almost wish I was going now,' she muttered, momentarily crestfallen.


Mr Hopkins looked casual but still very smart in his crisp white shirt with a black and grey checked tie, and a rather jaunty pair of burgundy trousers and matching waistcoat with large black buttons. I dawdled with Hermione at the side of the mint green and curdling cream coloured bus, counting the heads of children when their names were called by the headmaster as each stepped forward, handed him their permission slip and then boarded the bus. As the last of the youngsters from the local children's home got on, I heard a smart-looking officer's wife whisper 'gutter-snipes' to her companion. Hermione shot her a withering look and then boarded the bus herself, offering the children sweets from a paper bag. I noticed a look of deep admiration from the headmaster as he watched my colleague become firm friends with the children in less than a minute, making them laugh and swarm around her – each one eager to feel the glow of her irrepressible radiance.

Mr Hopkins began calling the names of his own pupils, who responded with practised compliance until he came to 'Colin Mires', when there was no answer. A brief look into the crowd of infants and juniors, then a shake of the head. Clearly this child's absenteeism wasn't a surprise

'Neil Bowyer, Jenny Bowyer,' the headmaster continued, unperturbed. Stacy's big brother and sister, I surmised, remembering the eventful Mums and Toddlers group earlier in the week. 'Tina Seaton, Karen Seaton' – both stepped forward. 'Kimberley Seaton' – no response. 'Tina, where's your big sister?' asked Mr Hopkins.

'Woodcraft Folk, sir,' answered the small brown-haired girl.

'Hmm, get on,' instructed the headmaster, frowning as he marked the register on his clipboard with a red X. 'Jennifer Wraight, Kevin Wraight,' he called.

A shy blond-haired boy, no more than six, squeaked, 'Our Jenny's gone to Woodcraft Folk too, sir.'

This time Mr Hopkins didn't say anything, but simply gestured his head towards the open bus doors. Relieved, the little boy sprang on.

'Donna Buss, Martin Buss, Kevin Buss.'

'Mr Hopkins, sir,' spoke up a sparky-looking girl in a red tank top and jeans.

'Don't tell me, Kevin's at Woodcraft Folk too?' retorted Mr Hopkins.

'No, sir, chess tournament, both him and Ian Bunyard,' replied Donna.

'Chess! He could barely play tiddlywinks during wet break as I recall,' challenged the headmaster.

'They're at a youth hostel with Scouts, sir,' perked up a smaller boy.

Mr Hopkins turned his dark eyes onto this child. 'Thank you, Brian Bunyard. Take Derek and get on the bus now,' he told them agitatedly, putting the lid back on his red biro.

I saw Ernestine Higgins walking up the hill in her midwife's uniform hand in hand with a lovely girl dressed in a yellow and white check cotton tunic with matching knee-length shorts and a blue denim jacket. A yellow ribbon shone in her beautiful black curly hair but she kept her large brown eyes on the pavement.

'Morning, Nurse Higgins,' I waved.

'Morning, Miss Hill,' puffed the midwife. 'I hope I can entrust my little Cecily to you on the school trip today,' she requested.

The girl gave me a shy smile.

'You can indeed. How old are you, Cecily?'

'I'm nine,' she replied quietly.

'Goodness me, you look so tall and grown up I would have thought you were at least 11,' I remarked.

'Onto the bus now, Cecily,' her mother instructed. 'You don't want it to go without you.'

We watched her mount the steps and then sit on the front seat alone.

'She's just started at St Agatha's,' explained Ernestine. 'She doesn't know the other girls yet.'

'Oh, was she in school in Maidstone before?' I asked.

Nurse Higgins nodded. 'I must be getting on with my rounds,' she said, looking at her nurse's watch.

The discerning adults now filed onto the bus too. I would have liked a roll call, as I wasn't entirely sure who everybody was, though I thought they'd gone overkill on the number of chaperones, which included me and Hermione, Mr Hopkins, the dishy vicar and half a dozen RAF wives. I'd wanted to sit with Hermione but she was on the back seat with the kids from the children's home and the handful of youth club members who'd actually turned up, leading a chorus of 'Bye Bye Baby' as the engine started and the radio came on, filling the bus with the sound of the Bay City Rollers. I had a double seat all to myself and was contemplating whether it would be above board to rest my eyes for a little while when Nick Shepherd squashed in beside me. His thigh pressed into mine. He seemed inappropriately close, as we'd barely been introduced. The smell of Old Spice and Head & Shoulders filled my nostrils. His curly hair was still wet at the tips and there was a waft of sandalwood. What do I smell like, I wondered, thinking back to last night and my late morning start. Brie, red wine and cigarettes from the pub. How disgusting and I don't even smoke. I tried to discreetly sniff my hair and took a polo mint out of my handbag.

As we were about to set off a cool blonde about my age pulled up next to the bus in a shiny orange Beetle and hopped onto the bus. She wafted down the aisle with only a hint of a smile in a lovely Laura Ashley dress and cream jacket and sat in an empty seat amongst the closed circle of RAF wives who'd positioned themselves a row away from the village children. One of the women waved to my brooding companion to come and join them and without a word he switched seats and sat next to the blonde, who rested a proprietorial hand on his knee and shot me a look of disdain. I slunk down in my seat feeling rather sheepish in my blue and red striped jumper and old jeans. But I was snapped out of my reverie by girls laughing – not jubilant but taunting – which pricked my ears.

'But where do you come from?' enquired Donna Buss as she

leaned over from the opposite front seat, putting her face right up to Cecily Higgins.

'I told you, Maidstone,' Cecily replied calmly.

'That's not what I mean. My mum comes from Maidstone and she's not a darkie. Where do you come from?'

'Maidstone,' replied Cecily once more.

'Are you taking the mickey?' challenged Donna. 'Because if you are, I'll give you a …'

Before she could finish her threat I was on my feet, heading to the front of the bus.

'Cecily, do you mind if I sit next to you?' I called. Parking myself in between the girls, I heard Cecily let out a sigh. She reached into her bag and pulled out a library book and found her place.

'I'm never sure whether I'm more of a Mildred Hubble or a Maud Moonshine,' I whispered.

She smiled. 'You're a Mildred,' she replied and continued reading her copy of *The Worst Witch*.

The only excitement Canterbury brought me was discovering a copy of *The Needs of Children* in a lovely bookshop. Cecily accompanied me around the cathedral and shops and I treated her to tea and cakes. It was a beautiful city to explore and we didn't lose any of the children. Even though Mr Shepherd didn't say another word to me all day, I chalked it up as a success.

Completely washed out at the end of Saturday's excursion I wanted nothing more than a hot bath and an early night. I'd only been in the tub about five minutes when I was again summoned by the flipping telephone.

'Hello,' I answered sharply.

'Country life not suiting you then?' I heard a familiar lilting Irish voice ask cheekily.

'Fiona, thank heavens it's you,' I said in relief. Glad to hear the wonderfully warm tones of my old nursing colleague and flatmate Fiona Lynch, now Flemming. It had been a year since she'd married the diligent, polite and lovely Dr Guy.

'Guy and I wondered if you fancied having a pair of weekend visitors?'

'Yes, please. When do you want to come?'

'Either the Friday night or Saturday morning of the weekend on 4 October, depending on shifts,' she told me. Guy was now a senior resident doctor and Fiona a theatre sister at Hackney.

'That would be lovely, please come.'

'Good. Guy's trying to persuade me some rural living would do me good. Expect gumboots, deer-stalking hats, tweeds – the whole kit and caboodle. It'll be hysterical,' she said, laughing.

And as I listened to her, I remembered that sometimes a long chat with a very dear friend can be better than a hot bath.

# 9

It felt wonderful to briefly bask in morning sunlight as I walked from the clinic down the hill towards Totley Brewery, which lay on the right side of the tracks next to the railway station. In the distance I could see farmers ploughing their fields, tiny squares on a patchwork quilt of fertile farmland and meadows, a striking mix of emerald, sapphire, amethyst and topaz crops so precious to the men and women who toiled on them. Ponies grazed on the long grass next to the children's playground hemmed in by hedgerows bowed low with the last of blackberries ripe for the picking. As I sauntered along I didn't mind being stopped every couple of minutes with cries of, 'I'm glad I bumped into you, Nurse. I wanted to ask you about ...' And even a 'Did you find that lettuce I left on your doorstep, Nurse?' I wasn't sure if some of Totley's residents had fully caught on to the free nature of the National Health Service; had they mistakenly left the produce in payment or was it an act of gratitude and friendship? I would have to consult Hermione and Mrs King on that.

I was almost knocked out of my reverie as I was crossing over the bridge at The Station Hotel. An orange Beetle came racing round the bend and hurtled over the small bridge without a moment's pause. I had to press my back into the low wall of the bridge to avoid being flattened. It left me feeling exasperated and unsteady on my feet. I took a moment's rest on a bench opposite The Station Hotel. The country inn was a square white building with six black painted windows at the top and five at the bottom, each with its own pink floral window box. Four wooden picnic benches stood unoccupied in the front yard, each with a large open blue umbrella with 'Totley Beer' written on in large swirly white letters. On the steps of the entrance were two enormous flower pots. All looked quiet and still at this time, with the occasional rumbling of a train coming into the station and then departing towards the coast or to Charing Cross. I couldn't imagine The Station Hotel was inundated with guests in this sleepy village and the lunchtime crowd was hours off.

I was surprised to see the Reverend Nick Shepherd emerge from the black front door of the hostelry. I wouldn't have taken him for a morning drinker, I thought. He didn't notice me standing agog on the opposite side of the road and walked quickly to his burnt-orange Marina. 'With those dark looks he's a bit like David Essex,' I mused. He didn't start the engine, but sat in the driver's seat, staring blankly into the distance and looking lost until he raised downcast eyes and caught me gawping. I felt uncomfortable; I'd lingered there longer than I'd meant to. I gave him a half-smile and walked on towards the brewery tithe cottages all the while squirming on the inside, feeling hot and flustered. I could feel my previously loose limbs tensing as I sensed him watching me scuttling away. A few moments later I heard the sound of an engine running smoothly behind me. Was it that orange Beetle returned to finish me off?

'Nurse,' I heard Nick Shepherd call to me.

I composed myself. I hadn't done anything wrong. 'Reverend Shepherd,' I answered.

'Nick, please. And may I call you Sarah?' I nodded. 'I wanted to ask you to dinner.' Now I was surprised. 'Can I telephone you?' I nodded again. 'Great, we'll talk soon,' he told me then sped off, leaving me in a stream of choking smog. Had I actually uttered more than his name? And now it would seem I sort of, almost had a date.

I cleared my head of thoughts of tall, dark and moody clerics as I waited patiently on the Bunyards' doorstep. No one home again? I pondered why and bit my lower lip. Of course Mrs Bunyard may have forgotten I was coming, it was easily done, but something in my gut told me she was avoiding me. I wrote out a little card.

Wednesday 1 October
Mrs Bunyard
Health Visitor called at nine o'clock. Will call again same
    time next week if convenient. If you've any concerns
    please call Totley Clinic.
Sarah Hill

After popping the note through the door I could have sworn I saw the upstairs curtains twitch. I momentarily moped. 'I should have come in my Mini; now I'll have to walk back up the hill feeling like I've missed something.' As I trekked up Station Road a woman in a white headscarf and huge sunglasses driving an open-top MG beeped at me, then waved and pulled over. It was Hermione.

'What you do think of my new motor car?' she called.

'It's smashing. What happened to your Mini?' I asked.

'Oh, I never stick to regulation vehicles. I was borrowing one while this baby was on order,' she explained, leaning over and opening the door on the passenger's side. 'Get in,' she told me enthusiastically. 'I need a hand with some hearing tests, Did you have anything scheduled for this morning?'

'I was going to get ahead on some follow-up visits but I don't have a primary visit booked in till this afternoon,' I answered.

'Who's got a new bundle of joy?'

'Valerie Milstead at Prospect Hollow in Fairy Woods.'

Hermione raised one eyebrow and frowned a little. I paused but she said no more. I jumped in and we sped off in her new MG. Hermione really is a law unto herself, I thought admiringly. 'Over 40 and still a real beauty. More like a movie star or a fashion model than a nurse – she should be gracing the cover of *Vogue* not up to her elbows in sore nipples and nappy rash.' I felt a little shabby sitting beside her and idly wondered why she had never married. She was such a catch.

'I hope you don't mind me stealing you? Mrs King was going to assist me with the hearing tests but she's had to attend an emergency case conference in Maidstone.'

'Not at all. Who are we seeing?'

'I've got nine tests to do this morning for mothers who can't get to clinic. They are rather stranded, I'm afraid,' Hermione informed me.

Nine tests! We'll be at this till midnight, I thought, but the first three went smoothly enough. It was fun being out with Hermione – she made everyone feel very special including me. As we drove along the narrow country lanes with the top down in the late morning sun my new friend told me, 'This is one of life's lovely moments,' and how right she was. The road ended abruptly and we trundled along the dirt track past a farmhouse towards the farm labourers' cottages way out at Hill Cott Farm.

'Now, Sarah. We're going to be doing a re-test for twin boys, Les and Alan Mires,' she explained. 'They're eight months old and failed their hearing test a few weeks ago. I'm still visiting Mrs Mires monthly and she is a nice woman but she is struggling – the boys still have their hospital name tags on – and she can't tell them apart yet.'

'Are they identical?'

'No.'

During our visits I couldn't help but feel there was a lot Hermione and Mrs King hadn't told me yet. More secrets, more glimpses into lives that didn't completely add up. I suppose she thought some of it I had to find out in good time and the rest of it was none of my business. I soon learned you cannot force a confidence and sometimes you wished you didn't have the keeping of them.

'Whose farm is this?' I asked.

'Mr and Mrs Baldwin. They are tenant farmers. I believe they've been on this land for over 50 years. I don't know how much longer they'll go on for – they lost all three of their boys. I believe they were privates in the Royal West Kent Regiment, very sad,' Hermione told me.

'They've no one to pass it on to, how sad.' I had a rush of feeling for my father and my lovely Uncle Jack from Stourbridge, who was married to one of my mother's many sisters. I knew he'd lived to never tell the tale of the Normandy Landings; my own father too had nearly died in India but you could only ever get the odd word from them on the subject. They didn't think they were heroes – they had simply survived. The scar of the men who never came back from the war was still here – they weren't forgotten by those forced to carry on without them; the empty place at the table was never truly filled again.

'Did you lose anyone in the war?' I asked Hermione.

'My father was a naval captain,' she told me. 'He went down with his ship.'

'I'm so sorry,' I apologised. Poor Hermione, what a terrible loss – she must have been only a child. 'That must have been very hard on your mother,' I sympathised.

'Etty has a very good pension. My brother was already at university, my older sister at boarding school and I went soon after but she kept my baby sister with her for company until she married 10 years ago.'

I'd heard Hermione talk about Etty. I'd been wondering all this time who she was but had been too polite to ask.

'You call your mother by her name?' I enquired.

'I told her when she came to live with me, Etty, we are going to be friends. Mother and daughter simply won't work. I couldn't have her thinking I was hers to order about,' Hermione informed me. 'She likes to try it on, though, but we all like our own way – I know I do. Still, at 84 I suppose Etty thinks she has everything to play for and nothing to lose,' Hermione said with a chuckle.

'Eighty-four?'

'Yes. She had two very late babies. I don't know what my father was thinking, putting her through that. It wasn't a kind thing to do. There was never any question of separate beds in our house.' Hermione raised her perfectly arched eyebrow once more.

As we came to the end of the dirt track Hermione was forced to park her MG in a side field before a level crossing that separated Hill Cott Farm from the labourers' cottages. I didn't have my wellies but luckily the ground was quite dry.

'Hello, Miss Drummond,' an older woman called as she walked over the crossing.

'Mrs Baldwin, how are you on such a lovely day?'

'I've been to drop a box off for Carol Mires.'

'Just the person we've come to see.'

'She's no better than she ought to be. Tell the girl to make things last and tidy up a bit, would you? I've left her a flitch of bacon, eggs and fruit 'n' veg but she'll have got through the lot by Thursday, you mark my words. She's not an ounce of thrift. She's sitting there right now making dresses. Radio blaring, TV chattering, children wailing, sewing machine roaring – it's a rubble of noise. Place is a tip, there are mouths to feed and she's wasting her time running up fancy little numbers. This generation, they don't know how easy they've got it.'

Hermione smiled but neither agreed nor disagreed – she was like a mill pond. 'I hope we see you at choir practice on Wednesday night,' she said, changing the subject.

'I've not missed one for 30 years,' replied Mrs Baldwin, a tad haughtily.

'Good for you, see you there,' Hermione called cheerily as we parked outside the end cottage.

The labourers' homes were plonked in the middle of a field. I could not believe my eyes at the sight of a young woman with a child on her hip pumping water into a bucket and then stumbling back to her house with the contents sloshing on her skirts.

'Have they no running water?' I asked Hermione in astonishment. She shook her fine head. There was a queue of women outside a leaky-looking old shed. I knew it would not be a potting shed or a tool shed but still I had to ask, 'Is that an earth closet?' Hermione gave a tiny nod and turned off the engine. It made Susan Bunyard's meagre accommodation look like The Dorchester.

We knocked at the end cottage, where the door was slightly ajar. I could hear the faint sound of 'Shang-a-Lang' by the Bay City Rollers coming from the kitchen. A small dark-haired girl dressed in a beautiful pale-blue smock with a blue ribbon in her hair was sucking her thumb, nose almost pressed up against a television set, watching *Play School*. The shock of this house with its peeling wallpaper and damp walls was outweighed by the surprise of there being a television set, and not any old telly but the very latest model. Not just a box but a TV unit with a Betamax videotape recorder as well. I'd only seen these in the shop windows of Harrods and Selfridges.

'Hello, Debbie, is your mummy in?' Hermione asked as she crouched down beside the child.

Debbie turned her head and smiled at Hermione and wrapped her little hands about her neck and gave her a cuddle. Hermione scooped up Debbie, giving her a good squeeze, and kissed the back of her head.

'Mummy get fire,' replied Debbie. She must have been at least three.

I looked around and noticed two good-sized babies lying on their backs on a large rug in front of a dwindling fire, their heads inches away from the unguarded fender, but before I had a chance to say or do anything, Mrs Mires stumbled in with half a pail of coal. It was a warm day and yet there was an undeniable chill in this cottage.

'Ah, Miss Drummond,' Mrs Mires called cheerily. 'What brings you here? We've run out of coal again and I don't have enough anthracite to keep the fire going,' she told us as she placed the pail on the hearth. 'Don't worry about the babies, they can't go anywhere. Not even rolling over yet. I said to my sister Judy it's a blessing in disguise, saves me a few months of running after them.'

'That's a lovely dress,' Hermione complimented her.

'Thank you. I ran it up myself last week.' She grinned and gave us a little twirl.

The skirt ballooned out of her scarlet princess dress. It had short puffed sleeves and a low round neck tied with a yellow bow and was covered with a smattering of blue and yellow confetti. She patted her rich brown hair flicked out at the bottom into place. Little Debbie wiggled out of Hermione's arms and helped herself to a cheese sandwich cracker out of an opened red packet of Ritz biscuits and returned to watching Johnny Ball.

'What can I do you for today?' asked Mrs Mires again.

'My colleague, Miss Hill, and I have come to re-test the boys' hearing,' explained Hermione. Mrs Mires stared blankly at her. Hermione walked over to the mantelpiece and picked up an unopened white envelope and gave it to her. 'I think this is the appointment letter, Mrs Mires. But not to worry. Is now a good time?'

'As good as any,' replied Mrs Mires, overly cheerful as she stuffed the still unopened letter into her dress pocket. 'Which one do you want first?' she asked.

'Les, please.'

Mrs Mires bent over her boys and stared at them hard. They kicked and gurgled at the sight of their mother but there was no babbling. 'Which one are you?' she asked one of her wordless children.

Hermione picked up the slightly larger of the twins.

'Look, this is Les,' she told his mother. 'See, he's got brown eyes, like yours.'

Mrs Mires stared into her child's eyes. 'Yes, that's right. Les from the Bay City Rollers has brown eyes too. That's who he's named after,' she told me proudly.

I picked up the other baby. 'And Alan has blue eyes,' I said. She gave him a quick glance and replied less enthusiastically, 'Like his Dad. Of course Eric Faulkner has blue eyes but Alan is my second favourite from the band.'

Baby Les fumbled with Hermione's green chunky beads and gurgled but he could not grasp them properly.

'Sit down on the sofa please, Mrs Mires,' instructed Hermione. 'Miss Hill, if you would distract the baby, please.'

I opened up Hermione's bag of tricks and took out her rattle, a bell and a teddy nestled in an assortment of multi-coloured bricks. Looking at Hermione you wouldn't expect this to be the contents of her bag, I thought.

'Would you like to play with these bricks, Debbie?' I asked softly.

The little girl looked at the toys in my outstretched hand briefly and shrugged. She picked herself up and walked straight out the front door. I must have looked a little taken aback as Mrs Mires told me, 'Don't worry, Nurse. She's going to use the outhouse.'

'Sit him up please, would you, Mrs Mires?' asked Hermione as she went behind the back of the sofa to begin the test.

Mrs Mires held her baby tightly as he kept flopping forward as soon as she loosened her grip to pat her hair or smooth her skirt.

'Would you mind if I turn the TV and radio off, Mrs Mires?' I asked.

'We always have that on,' she told me. 'But do it, if you think it'll help,' she acquiesced.

Conciliatorily, I turned the radio and the television right down and drew up a chair and sat opposite Mrs Mires and baby Les. I tried to distract him with the teddy while Hermione made a low noise with the rattle. The baby didn't turn round. Hermione made increasingly louder and louder noises but there was very little response. I rang the small handbell and offered it to the baby but he could not grasp it and it fell on the floor. It was the same story with the other twin. They both failed their hearing test again.

'I'll have to refer them to get their hearing tested by the paediatric consultant in Maidstone,' explained Hermione. 'It might be something like glue ear.'

'You don't think they are deaf, do you, Miss Drummond?' asked Mrs Mires. For the first time she seemed concerned.

'It is very difficult for us to test the babies' hearing when they can't properly sit or turn their heads very easily.'

'They are very big boys,' excused their mother.

'I'm also going to suggest they are checked for developmental delay.'

'What does that mean?'

'We want to know if there is a condition that is preventing them from responding and progressing or whether they need a bit more opportunity and stimulation,' Hermione tried to explain. Mrs Mires's face remained blank.

Debbie returned from her unaccompanied visit to the earth closet. Her baby brothers were back in their places in front of the silent television on a tartan rug. She turned the volume back up, then gave each of them a pinch and they cried. Then another little girl with the same dark hair and large brown eyes as Debbie, wearing a yellow smocked dress, skipped in and sat next to the other children on the floor. She picked up the teddy and righted the tipped-over cups, plates and biscuits and started to lay out a tea party while chattering away to herself. She would have looked exactly like Debbie if it hadn't been for the striking difference in their animation.

'Do you have another set of twins?' I asked Mrs Mires.

'She's my sister's little girl,' replied Mrs Mires sharply. 'They are only a fortnight apart.'

'Gosh, they look so alike they could be sisters.'

'Well, you're wrongtaking there, Nurse.'

'Good afternoon, Nicole. Where's your mummy today?' Hermione cut in.

'She's gone to work,' answered Nicole, clear as a bell. 'I miss her. But she says she'll be back to read me bedtime stories.'

'How lovely,' answered Hermione.

Nicole took a story book out of a rainbow-coloured backpack. It was *The Tiger Who Came to Tea*. She read it to her cousins. I was staggered, not just that this three-year-old child could read but that the twins and Debbie were both listening attentively – so, they could hear.

'What's for lunch, Aunty Carol? I'm hungry,' demanded bright little Nicole.

'I haven't got nothing in. Have some more Ritz cheese biscuits,' Mrs Mires told her niece.

'That's not proper food; that's a snack,' complained Nicole.

'Stop your yarping,' scolded Mrs Mires. 'Our Judy's bringing you up to be a right cheeky madam.'

'Didn't Mrs Baldwin leave a box for you this morning?' prompted Hermione.

'What am I supposed to do with all that? It's all odds and ends,' cried Mrs Mires, throwing up her hands in defeat.

'I could write you out some recipes,' I suggested.

'As if I've got time for reading blethering recipes with four kids to take care of.' I felt embarrassed for interfering and cross with myself. 'Our Judy will be here to pick up Nicole soon,' continued Mrs Mires. 'She usually brings me a loaf. I'm sure there's a tin of something in the cupboard. I've got no truck with making more work for myself with fancy cooking.'

'I'll send you a letter to arrange another appointment,' Hermione informed Mrs Mires as she packed up her bag of tricks.

'No need. You turn up when you like, Miss Drummond. We has difficulty ruggling about.'

'It must be hard,' I sympathised, trying to regain some lost ground. 'Is there no bus service nearby?'

'Are you taking the mickey? It's a two-mile walk to the nearest bus stop. And I only wear high heels,' Mrs Mires told me.

'I'm sorry. Of course it must be difficult to get out.'

Mrs Mires folded her arms and scowled at me. Hermione smiled kindly – I must have looked discombobulated. I didn't know quite what I'd done but I'd clearly made a complete pig's ear of this visit. 'That'll be another one who pretends she's out when I call,' I reproached myself.

The back door slammed open and a man with his sleeves rolled up and covered in grime stormed in. Mr Mires, I presumed.

'Is the lunch not ready yet, Carol? It's midday, for crying out loud,' he shouted, looking at the kitchen table which was awash with needles, thread, materials, buttons, ribbons and Mrs Mires's old sewing machine but not a scrap of food. 'You've been away with the fairies all morning again,' he sneered.

'No, the nurses have been testing the boys,' she protested.

'Never mind them. I need feeding. I've a ditch to dig this afternoon over at the top field.'

'You'll have to watch the kids while I go to the pump,' Mrs Mires instructed her peeved husband. He grunted and opened up his toolbox and sat at the kitchen table with his back to us as he shoved the haberdashery to one side and started to fiddle with some oily mechanical part.

'I'll see you out,' said Mrs Mires, showing us the door and following us out in the yard, pail in hand.

We said a strained goodbye to her as she waited in line at the water pump and despondently trudged back to the car in silence. Hermione started the engine but as I was buckling up I noticed someone small on the level crossing ahead.

'Isn't that Debbie Mires?' I asked Hermione, peering at the child walking on the railway tracks.

'I think it is. Come on, we'd better take her home.' Neither of us wanted to return to the Mires's house but we couldn't leave a three-year-old child wandering around on her own, never mind on a level crossing.

'She must have slipped out while Mrs Mires was getting the water,' concluded Hermione as we hastily trotted over.

'What are you doing out here, Debbie?' asked Hermione.

Debbie shrugged but accepted Hermione's hand as we walked her back home.

Hermione knocked on the front door still ajar from Debbie's escape. Mr Mires answered, a screwdriver in hand.

'We found Debbie wandering along the tracks at the level crossing. She must have slipped out,' explained Hermione as Debbie wandered back into her ramshackle home and took up her position in front of the TV.

'Are you busybodies telling me how to look after my own kids?' exploded Mr Mires as he waved the screwdriver in Hermione's face.

'What's all the shouting about?' called Mrs Mires, who came to the door in a translucent apron.

'These two interfering bloody women,' Mr Mires snarled in our faces.

'We'll be off now,' Hermione informed them as we turned and started to walk gingerly up the path.

'What are you doing? They'll report us to Welfare if you carry on like this,' Mrs Mires scolded her husband.

'We'll see about that,' puffed Mr Mires, charging at us, screwdriver still in hand.

'Run,' shouted Hermione.

We hurtled back over the crossing and sprinted to Hermione's MG. She rapidly reversed out in a cloud of dust to make a quick getaway but Mr Mires had caught up with us. He banged the bonnet of Hermione's sparkling new car with the screwdriver, leaving a huge dent. In fear of bodily harm Hermione put her foot down and we escaped down the track, leaving Mr Mires shouting obscenities and shaking his fists at us.

'Your beautiful new car,' I said, panting for breath and shaken.

'I'm sure Trev Bowyer at the garage will knock the dent out for me this afternoon if I ask nicely. Could have been worse. Could have been one of our heads,' Hermione said stoically. 'Never pick a quarrel, even when it's ripe,' she recited to herself.

'What?'

'Don't you worry, Sarah. When Mrs Mires finds out what he's done, he'll be lucky if he gets any hot meals for a fortnight.'

'What a horrible man!'

'Not a very savoury character. But Mrs Mires is really doing her best in very difficult circumstances.'

'Yes, those cottages are dreadful and in the middle of nowhere. With three children to look after not to mention her sister's little girl. She seemed very bright.'

'Yes. Judy Larkin, the child's mother, is a bright girl. She was only 16 when she had little Nicole. Sad to see wasted potential.'

'And is Nicole's dad around?'

'Oh yes, he's around.' Hermione paused, waiting for the penny to drop. 'You see, Sarah, the reason those little cousins look like twins is because they are half-sisters.'

As I followed the tractor tracks to Hollow Prospect that afternoon I was sorry to see clouds had invaded the sky and transformed it to a dishwater grey. The seventeenth-century smallholding could have been idyllic but it was a sad story of leaky guttering and missing tiles on the roof of an old stone barn that dominated the L-shaped farmyard. A couple of pigs grunted in a small sty too near to the kitchen door, hens scratched about at the water pump and a lone cow rested her head on the criss-cross gate. In the distance a tractor was ploughing the small field, preparing the earth for sowing the autumn crops. The barn door stood half open to reveal a dozen or so sheep bleating as they waited to be wormed before being moved out to pasture. A line of cloth nappies and white sheets fixed to the line with wooden dolly pegs flapped in the increasingly strong wind. There were no flower pots or a small herb garden near the kitchen door like Mrs Rudcliff had at Treetops, and though this tenant farm was far grander than the cottages the Mires inhabited it had the same haunted feeling, like you'd stepped back in time. It had been a beautiful house – in different hands Hollow Prospect would have been the sort of home Alex, my old flame from my Hackney days, had dreamed of living in.

The heavens opened and the rain came down in stair rods. A girl ran out from the farmhouse carrying a wicker basket and hurriedly starting taking the washing off the line. In moments her sky-blue tunic and jeans had a rising tidemark of rainwater. I rushed over to help her take the laundry in. We worked quickly and I followed her into the lean-to wash-house.

'Thank you,' she said breathlessly, putting the washing onto drying racks.

'You're welcome – Miss Milstead?' She nodded. 'I'm Sarah Hill, the health visitor.'

'Excuse the mess.' Her eyes rolled over the piles of laundry and dishes to be done. 'Only I have to do it all by hand and I've only this stupid old thing for hot water,' she explained, gesturing disdainfully at the old monster of a copper hopper over the wash-house sink.

'Gosh, that's hard. Especially with a new baby,' I sympathised.

'You don't know the half of it, Nurse. Well, you'd better come through.'

I followed her from the lean-to through to a big, chilly, dimly lit kitchen. The electric lights flickered as the rain rattled the panes of glass in the rotting window frames.

'As my uncles aren't in, we can use the parlour,' she informed me.

I was surprised to be shown into a very comfortable sitting room. Old-fashioned, yes, with the same mean little windows, but expensively decorated with fussy Victorian furniture and cabinets bursting with lovely ceramics and ornaments on doilies. I peeked into a cabinet – it was mostly hundred-year-old Wedgwood and Spode and not a chip to be seen. Two huge high-backed armchairs were placed on either side of an unlit fireplace with a footstool apiece. The kindling was laid out ready for the evening.

'We can sit here.' Miss Milstead ushered me to the only other seat, a hard wooden cushionless settle under the draughty window. Her baby was sleeping soundly, tucked into an old wicker basket very like the laundry basket we'd piled high with wet washing.

'He looks very peaceful.'

'For now, he is. It's a different story at night, I can tell you.'

'Have you decided on a name?'

'Michael.'

'That's a lovely name,' I cooed, placing a warm hand on his little chest. I felt the comforting rise and fall of his breathing and watched his lips pout and suck in his sleep.

'Dreaming of milk,' remarked his mother. 'Poor little chap.'

It felt nippier in the farmhouse than it did in the deluge outside. Valerie Milstead picked up an old crocheted blanket in different shades of green stripes and wrapped it round her tiny shoulders. Her face was pale, her hands chapped, and her hair was tied up in a faded blue headscarf. She was only 18, but already she had a worn and troubled air to her.

'How's your week going, Miss Milstead?' I asked, sitting next to her.

'I preferred last week when I was in hospital,' she replied. I smiled. 'They don't give me any rest,' she grumbled to herself.

'Your uncles?' I asked. She looked about us, and saw the tractor was still trundling along the wet fields and nodded. 'Mind you, they only really care about having clean shirts on market day. I bet before I came along they weren't so particular, and probably changed their shirts once a month,' she snorted. 'But the nappies, Nurse. They won't give me any money to get nappies and I've had to use these ancient cloth things. Poor little Michael,' she cooed over her sleeping baby. 'I feel all I do is wash and dry, and cook and tidy up all day long. And the baby screams and screams sometimes for hours, but I can't stop. I can't do it all.'

'Is there no one else to help you?'

Her eyes watered. 'My mum's dead. There's no aunties, or cousins or sisters. Just me and them.'

'Is the father here with you?'

She hesitated then replied. 'No, he was a boy I knew from the fairs. We aren't together anymore.'

'Did you grow up here?'

'No, I did not,' she replied indignantly. 'I grew up with my mum, in a very nice little council flat in Ashford.' She paused and I waited. 'She died two years ago. I had nowhere to go but here. I'd never even met my mum's older brothers before but they wrote me a letter saying I could come and live on their farm, and work in the house like my mum did when she was young. They made it sound very rosy. And look at the place! I never get to go anywhere or see anyone. They won't drive me and it's a six-mile walk to Totley and I don't even have a pram.'

'If we could arrange some transport would you like to come to one of the mums' groups in Totley?' I asked. After seeing Mrs Mires earlier I had an idea brewing.

'And have all those snooty women in the village look down on me, no thank you! And my uncles wouldn't let me go. There's too much skivvying to do here.'

'Are you a bit short on baby equipment?'

'You're looking at it. One tatty old basket, a few blankets and only the clothes I managed to knit myself, and I hate knitting. They've got big gappy holes in 'em.'

'If I could get you some clothes, maybe a pram and some nice second-hand bits and pieces, would that help?'

'Yes, Nurse, it would.'

'It might take me a few weeks to get it all together.'

'I'm not going anywhere, Nurse. Unfortunately.'

'How's the feeding going?' I asked.

'I breastfed him for the week we were in hospital but I'm not doing it in front of them. My boobs are like boulders at the moment,' she sighed, pressing against her breasts through the tunic. 'My National Dried is nearly out – could you bring me a few tins?'

'Yes, I could do. Have you got enough until I come again next week?'

'I suppose so.'

'Would the same time next week be convenient?'

'Could you make it a Tuesday? They often go to the market in Maidstone then.'

'Yes, I've got Totley baby clinic in the afternoon but I could come in the morning on a Tuesday. Would that suit you?'

'That would be fine, Nurse.'

When I left Hollow Prospect I had a list as long as my arm of things to see about for Valerie Milstead. As I ran to my Mini in the unrelenting rain the timeworn uncles were worming the sheep in the doorway of the old barn. I smiled and they scowled at me. Their niece returned to the wash-house and I watched as one of the uncles followed her in. I started to shiver, and it wasn't the rain.

# 10

It didn't stop raining for the rest of the week. I hovered in the doorway of Ivy Cottage overlooking my sodden garden, hoping the barrage of rain would stop but knowing it wouldn't. I'd stupidly left my umbrella in my Mini parked at the front and would now have to run through the muddy garden in my raffia wedge sandals – I'd left my wellies in the car too. It was already after six o'clock and Fiona and Guy Flemming's train was due in 10 minutes and I needed to pick them up from the station. I'd hoped to welcome my old Hackney hospital friends to my rural idyll with drinks in the garden before a delicious home-cooked meal. I'd also hoped I'd have enough time to wash and blow-dry my hair, put some make-up on, run round with the hoover and get dinner on the go but a call had scuppered all that.

I'd started work at seven o'clock in the morning so I could leave at 4.30 p.m. with a clear conscience, but when the phone rings at 4.28 p.m. on a Friday afternoon and you're the only one in the clinic you know you have to answer it.

'Hello, Health Visitors, Totley Clinic,' I answered.

'Miss Drummond?' cried an anxious voice down the other end of the line.

'Miss Drummond's out at the moment. It's Sarah Hill, can I help you?'

'Oh, it's you.' Followed by a pregnant pause. 'It's Carol Mires. Our Debbie's swallowed pennies and an old sixpence from my purse.'

'Is she choking?' I asked, worried the girl was turning blue as we spoke.

'No, it went straight down. I only know she did it because when I went to pay the milkman all my coins had vanished, the little madam. When I showed her my empty purse she confessed. Why would she eat them? Usually she's chomping down Ritz Crackers. I rang the doctors and that Dr Botten said I had to go to Casualty. I called 999 and as she's not choked or nothing they said it's not an emergency and they won't send an ambulance.'

'Oh, I see.'

'But I want her looked at – it can't be right having all those dirty old coins in her tummy. What if it does something to her? What if it kills her and I can't get to Maidstone Hospital because there's not a bus? Nurse, what if she dies?' Mrs Mires's anxiety was building until she broke into a high-pitched sob.

'She won't die, Mrs Mires. But I think you're right to want her to be seen by a doctor. Can no one give you a lift to Maidstone?'

'No one,' she snivelled.

I glanced at the clock. It was 4.30 p.m. 'I'll come out and give you a lift to the hospital,' I offered.

'Thank you, Nurse,' she sniffled.

Almost an hour later Carol Mires, her twins, cousin Nicole, little Debbie and me were waiting in Casualty, having arrived in my Mini – I now shudder to think of us all piled into the car like that.

The sister scolded poor Mrs Mires. 'You left your three-year-old unsupervised and she swallowed not one but several coins. You're lucky she didn't choke to death.' She looked at us all and continued. 'You can't all come through – what do you think this is, a circus? Only Mum and child to see Doctor, now.'

Carol Mires stood there open-mouthed, guilty and distraught.

'I'll wait with the children,' I told her.

She gave me a half-smile and followed the sister with Debbie in her arms. Her mascara was all smudged from our journey in the car from a mixture of heartfelt sobs and cries at her children to behave. Half an hour later, Mrs Mires returned with the sister, but minus Debbie.

'She's got to stay the night,' said Mrs Mires, shrugging. 'Can you give us a lift home?'

'Of course,' I replied, packing up the little ones.

'We should tell your health visitor,' the sister informed Mrs Mires. 'But we'll let you off this time, they're such dragons.' The sister chuckled to herself.

'Oh, are they indeed?' Mrs Mires turned on her. 'This is my health visitor. And I think she's bloody marvellous!', and she stalked off out of Casualty, a baby in each arm, with Nicole running after her.

Sister looked on aghast. I picked up my shoulder bag and bit my lip so I wouldn't laugh.

'I'll telephone later to see how Debbie's getting on,' I informed her. 'I promise not to breathe fire down the line', and I too followed Mrs Mires to the car park and drove them home.

By the time I got back to my little flat I only had five minutes to tidy myself up. I tried in vain to rub my hair dry with a towel and changed into some fresh clothes. As I came into the sitting room to pick up my car keys I reproachfully eyed my unpacked shopping on the kitchen table. 'You can't even get a takeaway in Totley – what will Guy and Fiona think after their long journey – not much of a welcome, is it?' I scolded myself. Before setting out to face the rain again I telephoned the hospital to see if Debbie had passed the coins. 'No change yet,' said the children's ward staff nurse, giggling down the telephone. Oh very, funny, I thought – it was exactly the sort of thing Fiona and I would have said during our Hackney days.

I made a run for it down the garden path but as I rushed through the gate onto the back lane I slipped and landed on my bottom smack into a muddy pothole. I could feel tears of exhaustion and frustration brewing inside me when I heard a friendly voice say, 'Can I lend you a hand, Nurse?' It was Clem stretching out a weathered hand to lift me up. He had a box tucked under one arm. I thanked him.

'Do you want to go inside and dry off?' he enquired gently.

'I don't have time,' I replied in a raspy small voice.

'Let me escort you to your vehicle then,' he said, offering me his steady arm, which I took gladly.

'What have you got there?' I enquired about the box.

'Apples from Mill Farm. They've got more windfalls than they know what to do with. I'm taking these beauties to make cider.'

'I didn't know you made cider.'

'Ay. And beer too. I'm taking these over to my store in that little hut opposite your garden. I've got bags of grain and boxes of apples to see it. It'll make for a very merry wassailing, come Twelfth Night.'

'I didn't know people still did that.'

'Oh yes. My Flo was the Wassail Queen.'

'Was she?'

'Oh yes. Lovely she was. I can still see her standing in the orchards over at Mill Farm on a frosty clear January eve and knowing she was the girl for me.' I smiled as I lost him for a moment to the memory of him and Flo in their courting days. He recited with such feeling:

Wassaile the trees, that they may beare
You many a Plum and many a Peare:
For more or lesse fruits they will bring,
As you do give them Wassailing.

'How lovely. It's a pity about all this rain. It'll make collecting the windfalls a bit dreary.'

'No, it'll clear tonight. Blue skies tomorrow.'

'You think so?'

'I do. You should take your guests down to Mill Farm and give them Londoners a taste of clean country living.'

'I couldn't do that.'

'Why not?'

'That would be scrumping.'

'I'll ask permission for you if that's what's worrying you. There'll be no problem there. He's a good chap, Sid Holleman. His farm goes all the way to the new Watermill Estate, past the station and on the other side of the train tracks. He won't miss a few apples.'

'If you're sure they won't mind,' I acquiesced.

'Not a bit. And you can use my little store to make your own cider if you'd like.'

'Oh yes, I would.'

'Do you know what to do?'

'Yes, my parents had orchards at our old house in Wales.'

Despite my dishevelled appearance I felt quite refreshed as we arrived at my Mini.

'Now, you have a lovely evening, Nurse. What are you serving your friends?'

'Oh, I don't know. I had an emergency and didn't get a chance to prepare dinner.' My face fell again as I remembered my unpacked shopping on the kitchen table.

Clem smiled. 'Well, true friends won't mind pitching in. Now you drive carefully, don't rush,' he instructed as he opened my car door.

Somehow I made it as the train was pulling out of Totley Station going onwards to the Kentish coast. My heart soared to see my friend, someone who'd known me since I was 17, Fiona Flemming neé Lynch, standing on the platform, a newlywed in her wide-necked red shirt and cream flares holding the handle of a neat little raspberry-pink travel case.

'Sarah,' she waved and called out my name. Her lovely lilting Irish tone was music to my ears as I ran down the length of the platform to meet them. I kissed Fiona on the cheek and then reached up on my toes to attempt to kiss Guy too, but fell short as he was over a foot above. He shyly arched down and kissed me on the cheek. His glasses were all misted over by the rain.

'Lovely to see you,' Dr Guy said, grinning at me.

'Quick, quick, get in the car before you're soaked to the skin,' I instructed them as we made a dash, shrieking with excitement as we ran.

'Haven't you got a fancy little run-around?' Fiona remarked, slipping into the back seat and pushing her long brown wet fringe out of her eyes.

'Perk of the job,' I said, beaming while I started the engine.

Guy got in next to me, his knees were up to his chin, and Fiona roared with laughter as we made the journey up the hill to Ivy Cottage.

'What delights have you got planned for us this weekend, Sarah?' enquired my friend.

'Well, if it's not too dull I thought apple picking, cider making and a home-cooked meal tomorrow night?'

'Apple picking?' repeated Fiona in surprise. 'It's a long way from our jaunts to High Street Kensington.'

'Is it too dull? We could go to Maidstone instead?'

'No, it'll be grand. Only Guy had his heart set on having a ride on a little train.'

'Didn't you just come on a train?'

'My grandmother used to take me on the Dymchurch Railway in the school holidays when I was a boy,' explained Guy. 'But really it was only a thought.'

'I'll see if I can find a timetable in the village shop. They usually have things like that – I'm sure we could squeeze it in.'

Guy beamed.

'Will the cider be ready for drinking in time for tomorrow night though, that's the real question?'

'No, but I know a man who has already made a bottle or two,' I replied, grinning.

As we made our way up to my little flat Fiona sniffed the air.

'Ooh, what's that delicious smell?'

I was perplexed. We arrived in the kitchen to discover the table was laid, the shopping put away and the oven was on. I peeked inside my ancient cooker to find a huge casserole was warming in the oven, wafting out welcoming smells for weary travellers.

'Sarah, a working woman and a first-class hostess,' Fiona congratulated me.

I was about to explain my huge failings on the home front when I noticed a little note on the kitchen sideboard:

Don't say a word. Our little secret.
Stew will be ready by 7.30 p.m.
Flo

I didn't breathe a word. God bless Flo and Clem! Coming to my rescue yet again. I smiled and took the undeserved compliment, pouring them both a glass of red wine. Guy disappeared to freshen up, I think discreetly giving us some girl time to catch up. Fiona spread out on my little sofa, kicking off her platform shoes and tucking up her feet underneath her as we prepared for a cosy evening. She opened her handbag and took out a packet of Consulate cigarettes. Lighting up, she asked me, 'So, what are the men like around here?' before taking a long drag and blowing smoke in my direction with a wry smile on her face.

'Non-existent,' I replied. 'You know health visiting doesn't have quite the same appeal as being in a nursing uniform with black stockings.'

'But having your own flat does make it a little easier than being in a nurses' home,' suggested Fiona coyly.

'I wouldn't want to get a reputation for gentlemen callers like those girls who had that flat before us on the Balls Pond Road,' I added and we both fell about laughing, remembering our shabby digs previously occupied by exotic dancers of some sort.

'All the men I meet are fathers, so they're all taken – mostly. Single women in the country don't get a huge number of invitations,' I continued, suddenly feeling quite lonely at the realisation that for over a month it had been mainly work, work, work and I hadn't even noticed.

'Oh, dear. I thought it would be all dashing squires like in Jane Austen,' teased Fiona.

'No, I've not been invited to dance at a single ball,' I said, smirking.

We were interrupted out of our girlish silliness by the sobering trill of my telephone.

'Hello,' I answered.

'Sarah, it's Nick.'

I paused. Who's Nick, I thought, and left an enormous gap of unanswered silence.

'Nick Shepherd,' further explained my caller. 'The vicar,' he added, a little peeved.

'Oh, Nick. Yes, sorry, hello.'

'We agreed I'd call to arrange a date?'

I supposed we did. 'Yes,' I muttered again, clearly dazzling him with my sparkling repartee.

'Could I take you out tomorrow night? Not in Totley. I was thinking we could drive to Whitstable. There's a rather good oyster place on the seafront.'

'Erm,' I failed to answer.

'Who is it?' hissed Fiona, leaning over the back of the sofa, agog with curiosity.

I covered the mouthpiece and whispered. 'It's the vicar. He wants to take me for oysters tomorrow night.'

'Ooh la la! Is he tall, dark and handsome?'

'Overwhelmingly so. But he makes me feel like an idiot.'

'Can't think why,' she mocked.

'Sarah, Sarah, are you still there?' Nick shouted, bringing me back to the conversation.

'Yes, sorry. Only I've got friends staying and er …'

'Ask him here for dinner tomorrow,' Fiona whispered.

'Would you like to join us here for dinner tomorrow evening?' I asked reluctantly. It hardly competed with a fancy meal on the coast.

'Yes, I'd love to. What time?' replied the Reverend Shepherd.

'7.30 p.m.?' I suggested.

'See you tomorrow night,' he finished.

'Yes …' but before I had a chance to say any more he'd hung up.

'You've got a date, then?' Fiona grinned jubilantly.

'I guess so,' I said weakly.

'Things are looking up, Sarah Hill,' Fiona told me knowingly, while topping our glasses up.

\* \* \*

Wiping the cobwebs off the barrels you could tell Clem's store was out of Flo's jurisdiction. A dusty dark place full of deep fermenting odours, spiders and mice droppings. Unlike the smells I associated with Flo Farthing's domain at the clinic of baking and coffee, beeswax furniture polish and disinfectant. No wonder she'd looked on in horror as Fiona, Guy and I entered the store with boxes of apples from a morning picking windfalls at Mill Farm. After the barrage of rain we'd had for the last few days it had crept in at the sides and one of the bags of grain had been soaked through, creating a special brew all of its own, bubbling over the edges in a golden brown stew and making the floor sticky.

'I'm surprised he keeps this place unlocked,' remarked Guy. 'Surely it's too great a temptation for the local teenagers, all this booze?'

'You're probably right. I've seen a few sneaking about at the witching hour down the lanes. Not much to do in Totley.'

As we'd made our way across the fields from the orchards at lunchtime groups of younger teens were emerging from their beds and congregating at the children's playground near the sports fields. It was a sad sight to see them occupying the climbing frames and monopolising the swings before they would move on to gather round the village shop before teatime. Not old enough to go out to clubs in Maidstone but too old for play. Some of my mums weren't much older and I realised places like Clem Farthing's store were probably used for much more than illicit drinking. Regretfully, it wouldn't be long before I was knocking on the door of some of those girls.

'Sarah, what do we do with this lot?' Fiona asked as she plonked her box of apples next to the cider press.

'Well, the basic rule is if we fill this barrel with four gallons of apples we'll get one gallon of cider. These windfalls are a super mix of Kentish apples. We've got russets, coxes and bramleys; we'll get a variety of honey and sharp dry flavours.'

'Ooh, aren't you the expert!' exclaimed Fiona with a chuckle.

'Not really, but I did used to help Dad in autumn half-term sometimes.'

'What about these few cooking apples and pears?' asked Guy.

'I'll use the pears to make a pear and almond tart for tonight. We can use the cooking apples to mix with the other varieties in the cider.'

'What's on the menu tonight, Sarah?' enquired Guy, his eyes widening.

'Clem told me I could have one of his chickens and Flo's picked a mountain of parsnips. I thought curried parsnip soup followed by coq au vin.'

'Very sophisticated,' said Fiona, grinning. 'Do you mean he's going to kill one of those hens we saw clucking in the yard this morning for our supper?'

'I think he wrung a few necks and dressed them on Thursday. Those hens in the yard have escaped for now.' Fiona's hands went up to her throat and she gulped. 'I know I feel the same. I can't look when he does it,' I consoled her.

'I've gone all goosepimply,' shivered Fiona.

'And you a theatre nurse,' I teased. 'Come on, let's roll out the barrel,' I instructed, changing the subject.

We chucked all the apples into the barrels and then crushed them up after dusting off Clem's old wooden cider press. We took turns to do the churning while the other pair watched on with a cup of tea and some homemade cake and sandwiches Flo had appeared with on a tray.

'She's such a mother hen,' observed Fiona, sitting next to me on an old work bench enjoying a cuppa as Guy took his turn at the press. Our clothes were stained with fizzy apple juices. Fiona sniffed her checked shirt. 'I smell like Casualty on a Saturday night,' she said giggling.

'Nearly over,' I said encouragingly. 'Flo lent me some bell jars and I sterilised them earlier. Once we've decanted this lot into them we're done.'

'When will the cider be ready?' asked Fiona.

'In about six weeks.'

'Who's going to be your slave labour next weekend?' she enquired with a raised eyebrow. 'Maybe it'll be your dark dreamy parson.'

'I don't think he's the type to get his hands dirty. And he's not *my* anything,' I scolded my friend with a light touch of the ribs.

'If you say so, Sarah. It'll be your birthday in six weeks. Sounds like a good excuse for a party.' Fiona was right. But who would I ask? It's not like I had any close friends in Totley yet. 'Penny for them?' she probed.

'It's nothing. In retrospect it was easy at Hackney. There was always someone to pal up with, always something going on. I'm still adjusting, that's all,' I brooded.

'Life moves on.'

'It does. It's not that I'm unhappy. I love it here, it's just …'

'It would be nicer if you had someone to share it with,' and she squeezed my hand. We both knew I was thinking of Alex. He would have loved Ivy Cottage, the garden and this – doing exactly this.

'Is Maggie Appleton coming to visit you soon?'

'I hope so. Only we haven't fixed a date yet.'

'I haven't seen her around much but then you hope you won't see any of the little ones from Infants Ward in theatre, don't you?'

'I suppose they go to Great Ormond Street.'

'Didn't you want to do paediatrics there?'

'I did at one time. But I do think health visiting is the right choice for me. But it's overwhelming. Most of the time I don't know what I'm doing. I'm listening, observing, trying to be helpful and not say or do the wrong thing. It's a minefield every day. You'd think it'd be simpler in the country, but it's not. It's just less obvious. All behind closed doors.'

'What are your colleagues like?'

'They're wonderful – mainly. There's one dipsomaniac doctor and one besom of a health visitor ...'

'Aren't there always.'

'I don't know how they know so much. They're so wise and calm and fun actually. Despite the age gap they're lovely to be with.'

'Motherly?'

'Very motherly. But not like my mother, not a bit.'

Guy finished churning the last of the cider as Clem appeared in the doorway.

'I've popped the poultry up to your flat, Nurse,' he called.

'Thank you so much, Clem.'

'I've come to see if you needed a hand. That last bit lifting the barrels is heavy work.'

'Mr Farthing, if you wouldn't mind helping me, we could let these two ladies make a start on getting ready for this evening,' suggested Guy.

'That's what I was thinking, Dr Flemming,' replied Clem.

Fiona jumped down off the old table and kissed Guy on the cheek. 'You're both mind readers. I could do with a lovely long soak in the bath while Delia Smith makes a start on the dinner,' she said, winking.

* * *

After dinner Fiona fired up the old Dansette record player I'd bought on an outing with her to Portobello Market at the beginning of my nurse training. Her fingers ran over it nostalgically. It felt like only yesterday that I was a teenage student nurse, uncertain whether I'd even make it through training, and now here we were in our twenties having a dinner party. Fiona lifted the needle and put a record on. It was David Essex's 'Hold Me Close'. I'd bought it on the trip to Canterbury the previous weekend. Nick Shepherd refilled my glass with Clem's homemade cider. Goodness, it was potent – we were all absentmindedly swaying to the music.

'I think I've probably had enough,' I said to Nick.

'Let's live a little,' he said, grinning, his dark eyes twinkling. As I've said, he looked a bit like David Essex, only posher.

'You look like you're far away,' he said, touching my elbow, with a steadying hand.

'I was thinking how quickly time goes. One minute you're a student full of dreams living in the big city and the next you're in a respectable responsible job in a tiny village where if someone broke a window it would make the local headlines.'

'I know what you mean,' he nodded. 'It's like your whole life has been mapped out for you and you don't even know if it's what you want.' I wasn't sure if that was what I meant but I didn't want to interrupt. 'Do you believe there's one right person for everybody?' he asked. If there was what hope was there for me? I'd found and lost him already, I lamented. Taking a big drink of my cider I lost myself for a moment in the huge dark eyes of the brooding vicar. 'If you'd found them you'd know, wouldn't you? You wouldn't have doubts?' he continued.

Surely he couldn't be talking about me? 'I think you'd know,' I replied. This conversation felt a bit ridiculous. I wrinkled my brow in concentration.

'Oh, so do I, Sarah, so do I,' he gasped. 'But sometimes you meet people and they are so sure and you just go along with it because it all looks right on paper. But there's no, no …'

'Spark?'

'Yes, spark. And everything is so polite. So nice, so orderly and you find yourself so bloody bored.'

I really didn't have any idea what he was banging on about. I smiled and nodded sympathetically. He refilled both our glasses with cider. Fiona and Guy were cuddled up in the corner.

'They look happy,' Nick observed.

'They're well suited,' I agreed.

'But not the same?'

'Not on the paper perhaps, but they complement each other. They have a deep regard for each other, I think.'

'That's it. Your opposite, not your twin.' He'd lost me again. 'I knew you'd understand,' he exclaimed.

Irreverently he put his arm around my waist and we danced closely together. He was strong, and warm and comforting. I placed my head against his chest and it felt nice to lean on someone. To not be alone. Nick lifted my chin and looked into my eyes, searching for something. Then he kissed me so hard he nearly knocked me backwards. It didn't feel like passion, it felt filled with longing and desperation and far too much of Clem's scrumpy.

There was a huge crash outside and he sprang back from me, his eyes overly bright and panting for breath. I rushed to the window. Someone was in Clem's store at the bottom of the garden. It was so dark in the unlit garden that we could only make out a shambling figure heading towards Ivy Cottage, eventually banging into the back door. Fiona and I jumped with every bang.

Fiona fearlessly opened the window and leant out to give them a piece of her mind. 'Who do you think you are, making all that racket?'

There was no reply. A shadowy figure was on their hands and knees knocking at the door before collapsing onto the ground. Making huge grunting snore-like noises.

'It's probably some legless local lad,' suggested Guy. 'Better go and check they haven't hurt themselves.'

We crept down the stairs to my backdoor, Guy with his doctor's bag in hand. He opened the door and the intruder fell at our feet. It was an enormous inebriated badger.

Nick started to laugh and we joined him in relief as the badger drunkenly snored in my porch. A torch beam shone in our eyes. We could hear footsteps coming down the garden path.

'What have we here then?' asked Clem, followed by Flo.

'Oh my Lord,' cried Flo. 'Not again. I told you to lock up that store, Clem Farthing,' she scolded. 'I'm so embarrassed. You've ruined Miss Hill's dinner party. What will her friends think? Oh, and hello, Vicar, I didn't know you were here.'

'Good evening, Mrs Farthing,' replied Nick, attempting a sober voice.

'It's not Clem's fault,' I soothed.

'It most certainly is. I said to him to get rid of that fermented sack of grain. The badgers are mad for it. Look at the havoc. Who else has sloshed beasts roaming in their gardens at night, I ask you? You get your wheelbarrow, Clem Farthing, and take that creature to the wood to sleep it off.'

Guy looked at Nick and they started to roll up their sleeves.

'Don't you help him,' Flo instructed firmly. 'He's got to learn his lesson. Go back to your evening, in with you,' she shooed us back indoors.

All four of us looked pityingly at Clem.

'I'll be all right. You young folks enjoy your party. I'll bring you another bottle of my cider, that'll see you right.'

We couldn't stop laughing for the rest of the evening. I must have dozed off because I woke up at about three o'clock in the morning with my head on Nick's shoulder as he snored next to me on the sofa. Fiona and Guy had made it to bed. I nudged him.

'Nick, wake up. It's three in the morning.'

'I'll sleep on your sofa – it's OK, I don't mind,' he replied groggily.

'*I* mind. What'll people say? Come on up, back to The Parsonage.'

'I hate The Parsonage,' he protested.

'How can you say that? It's a beautiful house.'

'It's dull. My life is dull,' he howled.

'Come on, it's the drink that's made you maudlin. Now come on, get up.'

'You make me feel a little brighter,' he informed me, turning on that big smile of his.

'We barely know each other,' I informed him, dragging him to his feet. After putting his coat on I led him a step at a time down the stairs.

'Don't cast me out into the dark,' he cried absurdly.

'Oh, don't be so bloody dramatic.' I opened the door. Then I had second thoughts. 'Are you all right to walk home?'

'Madam, are you insinuating that I am drunk?' he asked pompously. Where was Mr Cool now?

'We're both tired. Have a big glass of water before you go to bed,' I ordered, patting him on the back as he crossed my threshold.

'Will I see you tomorrow morning?'

'It *is* tomorrow morning.'

'No, at church?'

'Maybe, why?'

'It's harvest festival.'

'Yes, all right,' I settled.

128

I shut the door firmly and leant on it for a moment, breathless with the exertion. I could hear a beautiful tenor voice singing 'Hold Me Close' as he made his way home. Of course he could sing but what on earth was he playing at? I wasn't sure if it was a sin to not keep a promise to a vicar but I felt certain he'd have a sore head and a heart full of regret in the morning. I didn't even know if he liked me, and did I like him? Was it just making the most of a very small pool? Maybe tomorrow we should duck out of church and go straight for a jaunt on the Dymchurch Railway instead. But when I suggested this to Fiona and Guy at breakfast over eggs and bacon, Fiona wasn't having any of it.

'Certainly not, we're very keen to see the Reverend Shepherd in action, aren't we, Guy?' And that was that. At ten o'clock I had Flo on one side and Fiona on the other in a pew in St Agatha's Church.

In the front row I noticed Mrs Bourne with her two girls. She was shifting uncomfortably on the hard wooden bench, her hand on her pregnant belly. Next to her was that smart blonde from the school trip.

I whispered to Flo, 'Who is that?'

'Miss High and Mighty in the peach suit?'

'Yes,' I confirmed.

'That's Felicity Bourne. Her dad's a bishop and her brother is that one serving on the altar now with the fair hair.'

'Diane Bourne's husband?'

'Yes, she's a pretty girl, isn't she? They live at Kings Manor on the Malling Road. Big posh house and her and those girls are always dressed beautifully. He works in London during the week – he's some big wig at a university – so we only see him on Sundays. They're a very holy family.'

The service started and it was sweet to see all the children come in with their offerings. I'd been christened Nitty Nora by a few of them after my school-nurse visit to the infants at the beginning of the week. Little Jenny Bowyer told me how she hated harvest festival as the other kids in her class always brought in huge fruit baskets wrapped in cellophane and ribbons for their offerings and her mum always sent her with a tin of Heinz tomato soup. With Mrs Bowyer's permission I'd baked a loaf of a field mouse in a field of corn and given it to Jenny to take up. I watched her beam with pride as she made her way up to the altar and was told to put it in pride of place right in the middle. At the end of the service Trev and Jackie Bowyer came to see me.

'I think I'll have to bid for that loaf at the auction. Our Jenny doesn't want anyone else to have it,' Trev Bowyer said, chuckling.

'I'm glad she likes it.'

'Likes it, she's as pleased as punch,' added her proud mother. 'You'll have to teach me to bake like that.'

'Well, I have been thinking about starting a mothers' interest group,' I suggested.

'What's that?' asked Mrs Bowyer.

'We'd get together once a week and do stuff. Like baking, or making presents, or learning about first aid or a trip to the zoo or something. But only if the mums want to.'

'Would it cost anything?'

'No, it would be free. I'd see if I could get a little bit of money for the materials and ingredients and even the tea and coffee would be free. Anyone could come. It would be a chance to get together and learn how to do a few nice things for the family on a budget.'

'That sounds like a great idea, Nurse. I'll spread the word.'

'Thank you. It's a pity the mums out on the farms can't come. There's no bus.'

'There used to be a clinic bus.'

'Did there?'

'Oh yes. The council laid it on. But they stopped doing it a while back.'

Now there's a thought, I pondered. A bus not only to Totley but for the mums nearer The Meadows, like Carol Mires. I would talk to Mrs King and Miss Drummond tomorrow.

Fiona and Guy wandered over. 'Shall we say goodbye to Nick?'

I glanced over but he was still outside the church doors, talking to the Bourne family.

'He looks busy.'

'Oh come on, scaredy-cat,' she teased, tugging my arm.

'Good morning, Nurse, Dr and Mrs Flemming,' Nick formally greeted us. 'Have you met Mr and Mrs Bourne and Miss Bourne?'

'Hello, Miss Hill. It's nice to see you,' responded Diane Bourne.

Her sister-in-law continued loftily. 'I said to Father the new houses will completely spoil the character of the village.'

'People need decent homes, Felicity,' Nick interjected.

'What about those sweet little cottages by the brewery? They're perfectly charming. Not some modern monstrosity.'

'Have you ever been in one of those sweet little homes?' I asked.

'Heavens, no.'

'They don't have an inside toilet or hot running water.'

'I dare say they are used to it,' she sniffed.

'I think many of my mums' lives would be much easier if they had a modern home with indoor plumbing and a washing machine.'

Nick grinned at me. 'The lorries are a worry, though. The developers have promised not to go through the village to keep disturbance down.'

'We must be getting off. Enjoy your Sunday,' I ended the conversation.

Fiona, Guy and I wandered back through the churchyard. As we reached the gate, Nick came rushing up behind us.

'I wanted to say goodbye properly. It was lovely meeting you, Fiona and Guy. Such a fun evening,' he said with unusual warmth, shaking their hands. 'Sarah, are you free on Friday?'

'Well, I'll have to check my diary.'

'Maybe we could try out that restaurant in Whitstable?' he suggested.

'It's such a long drive and I never know what time I'll get off. What about a drink in The Good Intent instead?'

'All right, I'll telephone you,' he said, waving as he made his way back to the church.

'Are you playing hard to get?' Fiona asked me.

'No, it's not that. But it does feel like being a pawn in someone else's game,' I sighed.

# 11

I was going to be a bit sneaky. Susan Bunyard was clearly avoiding me – but why? I needed to know she was all right. Baby Sharon's six-week check was due in a week. I decided to knock on Mrs Bunyard's door at nine o'clock to book her in. The first few cottages in the row opposite the brewery were caked in reddish-brown dust and I quickly saw why, as a lorry bound for work at the new Watermill Estate rumbled through the village, leaving a dust cloud in its wake.

'They're supposed to go round the village,' the postman grumbled at me. 'I'm going to get onto Reverend Shepherd, he's on the parish council. They need to read them developers the riot act.' And he marched off in the direction of St Agatha's, I assumed to do just that.

The milk van trundled past, my milkman waving as he passed by. 'Morning, Nurse,' he called. 'I've left you two pints and some yogurts, so don't leave 'em too long on the doorstep.'

I knocked on Susan Bunyard's door. A pair of red eyes in a pale face creeped around the door.

'Good morning, Mrs Bunyard. I wanted to see how you and baby Sharon are. Is now a good time? Do you have visitors?'

She shook her head, 'No, Nurse. You'd better come in. I've fed the baby, she's having a nap.'

I followed Mrs Bunyard through to the kitchen. What's happened to her, I thought, a string of possible scenarios racing

133

through my mind. I watched cautiously as she agitatedly moved about, unable to settle; reaching for a cup from the cupboard then turning to put things away from the draining board, before hunting for a spoon – leaving every task incomplete. She kept her back to me, her hands constantly reaching up to her face, wiping her eyes. I notice an opened re-directed envelope on the sideboard stamped HMP Pentonville. Susan Bunyard turned round and saw me glancing at the envelope. She snatched it up and crushed it in her hands.

'You nosey parker,' she cried before breaking down into a torrent of tears.

I pulled out a kitchen chair and she crumpled onto it, her head in her hands, heaving huge sobs. I stood next to her, my hand pressed lightly on her shoulder until the crying stopped. She reached up and touched my hand with just her fingertips and quivered.

'I'm sorry, Nurse.'

'Do you want to talk about it?' I asked.

'If I tell you, will you keep it a secret?'

'Of course I will,' I confirmed.

She sighed and all the breath flowed out of her in a forlorn raspy little moan. After fetching her a glass of water I sat next to her, resting my hand on top of hers and waited. She eventually flattened the envelope onto the kitchen table in front of us, pulled out a letter written on blue lined paper and smoothed out the creases. It was poorly written in pencil and lots of the words had been censored in cruel black strips.

'I was taking the milk in and the postman took the opportunity to cross the lane and hand me this letter. I could see the prying, smirking look on his face. I took it from him and shut the door. But I peeped through the nets and he was talking to the milkman. It'll be all over the village by lunchtime. And what will my Alan say?'

'It's only a letter, it doesn't mean you've done anything wrong. We've no control over the letters we receive.'

'Oh, but I *have* done something, Nurse. This letter, it's a visiting order from Charlie Carter.'

'Who's Charlie Carter?' I asked. But I already knew. Thinking back to the birth, her quick delivery and the moments before she'd had little Sharon, grasping my hand and begging me, 'Whatever happens, don't let them take the baby away, please.' Her panicked face and that request had been at the back of my mind ever since.

'He's my biggest mistake,' replied Susan Bunyard. I waited for her to find the words. 'I was only 16. I'd just lost Ma. I met Charlie, got pregnant and when I was seven months he got caught red-handed, nicking a telly from the neighbours, and he had her purse in his pocket as well. I know now he was bad 'un; money was always going missing from my purse, and little things like my parents' silver candlesticks from when they were married and a Wedgwood jug my ma loved suddenly vanished from the mantelpiece. It wasn't even the first time he'd had his collar felt – he'd been up before the beak a couple of times already so the judge sent him down.

'I didn't know what to do. My dad's older sister, Aunty Mildred, said the best thing was for her to have the baby, so Michelle wouldn't have the shame of having an unmarried mother and a convict for a father. And I agreed. God forgive me, I agreed. But I couldn't bear not seeing her, not being able to tell her I was her mum. After her first birthday my aunty wouldn't even let me visit, said it was too confusing for Michelle. And my dad was so lost after Ma died, he didn't say a word. When I met Aly it seemed like a good opportunity for a fresh start. But now Charlie's gone and stirred it all up again. He didn't know where I was so he sent it to Aunty Mildred's house and she sent it on, but I can tell she's opened it and read it. What does Charlie want from me? I can't make head nor tail of it from this letter.'

'Do you want to see him? You don't have to go if you don't want to.'

She paused. 'I do. He's Michelle's dad. I haven't seen him for so long. There's things I never got to say. I never told him I gave Michelle away. He'll be so angry.'

'Never mind him. What about you?'

'I want to see him, I do. I need to tell him. It's such a weight. I worry all the time. But I don't want Alan's family to know. They already think I'm not good enough. What if they take Sharon away too?'

'No one's going to take Sharon away from you.'

'No?'

'You're a very good mother.'

'You think so?'

'Yes, I do. When is the visiting order for?'

'This Thursday, the ninth. How am I going to get to Pentonville? I don't have the money for the fare. I'd have to ask Aly and then he'll want to know why. I can't tell him, I can't tell him.'

'If you want to go, I can arrange transport for you to London.'

'Really, you can do that?'

'Yes, I can. Would you like me to?'

'Yes, Nurse. I've got to go, I don't know why but I need to see Charlie.'

'Leave it with me, Mrs Bunyard. I can arrange transport to get you to the prison. We don't need to tell anyone if you don't want to.'

'Thank you, Nurse,' she clutched my hand and we sat in silence for a while, letting it all sink in.

\* \* \*

When Community Transport rang to confirm they could take Susan Bunyard to Pentonville I was in my Mini en route to the clinic after visiting Valerie Milstead while her uncles were out of the way at Maidstone Market. I'd raided the cupboard for National Dried Milk for her baby. Miss Milstead thought it was free and I didn't have the heart to tell her it wasn't; for the next four months I ended up putting the money in myself whenever the milk clerk cornered me about stock being unaccounted for. Regrettably, it was Mrs Jefferies who answered my call from Community Transport; Tuesdays being one of the days Nitty Nora graced us with her presence. As I walked into the health visitors' room Mrs King was writing up her notes and Mrs Jefferies was sitting on my desk on *my* phone.

'Well, she's a slip of a girl. She really doesn't know about these sorts of people. Boarding-school jolly hockey sticks type. They'll be pulling the wool over her eyes. Did she give a reason?' Mrs Jefferies glanced up, clocked me, turned her back to me and continued. 'I really wouldn't bother, it's a waste of public money. Goodbye,' and she hung up and continued sitting at my desk, looking over it for clues.

'Were you talking about me?' I asked, quaking with supressed anger.

'Yes,' she answered without looking up.

'Who to?'

'Community Transport. I told them not to bother. There's a charge, you know. We're health visitors, not a taxi service. The girls round here have got legs, haven't they? They can walk. Who was it for, anyway?'

'Firstly, how dare you disparage me to another organisation like that, it's completely unprofessional. Secondly, you've got no right to be cancelling it when you know nothing about the client or their situation. Thirdly, I'm not telling you a thing about it for fear it'd be broadcast to anyone who happens to phone the clinic. So, you can get your bum off my desk while I phone Community Transport to tell them we absolutely will be needing their service, and I'll be paying for it myself so it has nothing to do with you or anybody,' I finished telling her and swept into my chair and picked up the phone to confirm the booking.

'Well, I've never been spoken to like that in my life,' huffed Mrs Jefferies. 'You're a silly girl,' and she gathered up her handbag and coat and flounced out of the office and didn't return until the following week.

'Miss Hill,' called Mrs King.

I looked up, waiting to be reprimanded. 'Yes, Mrs King,' I answered weakly, my adrenalin rush now over.

'Next time you wipe the floor with Mrs Jefferies would you warn me first, as I'll put on my tin hat,' she said with a laugh.

Susan Bunyard was on my mind all week. By Friday morning it felt like the clock was ticking by very slowly as I waited until I could be sure Alan Bunyard would be at work, giving me an opportunity to pop in and see how she was after visiting Charlie Carter at Pentonville. I occupied myself with calls to the local authority to see about reinstating the bus for the mothers from the farms and labourers' cottages who couldn't get to the clinic. We reached a compromise that the bus would run every Tuesday afternoon for Totley baby clinic and once a month on Thursday mornings for the clinic at The Meadows, a council estate miles away in the middle of nowhere on the outer edges of Malling. The Meadows had a social club, a small parade of shops and a GP's surgery which hosted the baby clinic. The previous GP had gone before I came to Kent and the post remained unappealingly vacant with an array of locums filling in. It wasn't an adequate transport service by any means but it was a start. I was excited the authority also said yes to trialling a bus service for my proposed Mothers' Interest Group on Monday mornings on a temporary basis into the church hall at St Agatha's and back, depending on the uptake. Nick Shepherd had given me carte blanche to use the room gratis as it was deemed a community activity and I'd decided I would fund the group myself for now. If it worked I'd then talk to our manager, Miss Presnell, as Mrs King and I had decided it was easier to say 'yes' to a successful group than to an idea about one. We'd agreed with Hermione not to mention it to Nitty Nora until it was necessary, as we were certain she'd object out of spite and try to scupper the group before it had even begun.

I fetched the typewriter and typed out a list of activities for the group to do between now and Christmas. The slow clattering noise filled the office broken by long pauses when I hit the wrong key and was forced to reach for the Tipp-Ex more than once.

WEST KENT HEALTH AUTHORITY
MOTHERS' INTEREST GROUP
Meetings 9.30–11.30 a.m. Mondays in St Agatha's Church
    Hall, Totley.
13 Oct. 1975 – Presentation, rota and funding. Discuss ideas
    for trips and activities
20 Oct. – Jam and preserves
27 Oct. – Half-term
3 Nov. – Pickles
10 Nov. – Sewing bee
17 Nov. – Christmas cake
24 Nov. – Christmas cards
1 Dec. – Christmas decorations
8 Dec. – Christmas shopping to Maidstone on bus
15 Dec. – Christmas party

I pulled the finished plan off the typewriter with a satisfied swoosh. The office was empty and I felt my enthusiasm bubbling over. I needed to share this with someone – my fingers started dialling, the rotary dial spinning back infuriatingly slowly as my eager digits turned each number.

'The Parsonage, Totley,' answered the smooth voice.

I could not bring myself to call him Father Nick – it was too discombobulating.

'Hello, Reverend Shepherd. It's Sarah Hill,' I said, still unsure of our level of intimacy.

'Yes, I know,' he replied warmly. 'You aren't ringing me to complain about the lorries going to the Watermill Estate too, are you?'

'No, but now you mention it.'

'The developers have given me their word there'll be no more traffic through the village from next week. They'll take the long way round across Fairy Hill and use the service entrance down the farm track. Problem solved,' he concluded triumphantly.

'Well done,' I praised. 'I wanted to tell you I got the go-ahead for the bus and it'll be free to pick up mums from 13 October to bring them to the church hall, if that's still OK?' I told him in a rush of enthusiasm while attempting to maintain my professional tone. I could hear the amusement in Nick's voice.

'Yes, that's fine by me. But, Sarah, the 13th is this Monday.'

'Yes, that's right,' I answered.

'Today's Friday. How will you get it arranged in time?' he queried.

'Oh, heck! I don't want to ring back and say I made a mistake before it's even started,' I admitted.

'We can do a few leaflets to hand out in church on Sunday and I can make an announcement after my sermon,' he suggested.

'Would you do that for me?' I was pleasantly surprised.

'Yes, of course.' He was much more sincere than usual. There was less chat and more friendliness. I preferred it to the smooth talking that always left me feeling on the back foot.

'Thank you. I'll ring up a few of the mums.'

'Great plan. You only need a few to get it started.'

'What if no one comes?' I pondered, momentarily deflated once more.

'If you build it they will come,' he said with a chuckle.

'No, really. What if no one wants the bus or the group?' Self-doubt now crept in, bursting my bubble of optimism.

'I'm sure a few people will come, if only for a free cuppa and a biscuit.'

'Oh, thanks.'

'Trust me, people will go out of their way for a free biscuit.'

'Nick,' I started and then paused, not knowing what I wanted to ask him.

'Less chat. More phoning,' he instructed, filling the gap in the conversation. 'If you tell a few mums it'll spread like wildfire by pick-up time.'

'All right,' I concurred.

'Don't forget you promised you'd spend the evening with me at The Good Intent.'

'I won't,' I replied slightly absentmindedly, already making a list of mothers to telephone in my head. Flo bustled in with a yellow duster and lemon Pledge. The spray started to tickle my throat and I could feel a coughing fit coming on.

'Seven o'clock and don't be late,' Nick reminded me once more.

'See you later,' I said, very primly aware Flo's ears were pricked up.

'Goodbye, Nurse,' he responded with mock formality.

'Reverend,' I countered, putting my finger on the button and redialling. 'Hello, Mrs Mires. I've got some news …' I started.

After the lunchtime break was over at the brewery I was hopeful Susan Bunyard would be home alone. I stood once again on the doorstep of her cottage praying that yesterday had turned out well. The familiar peeling red-painted door was opened not by Mrs Bunyard but her fatigued husband. He had bloodshot eyes and was wearing crumpled flared jeans and a striped T-shirt, not his usual ale-coloured work overalls. Baby Sharon was in his arms – he rocked her back and forth with a steady hand.

'Mr Bunyard,' I said brightly with a slightly strained smile.

'You'd better come in, Nurse,' Alan Bunyard invited me in with a furtive glance up and down the row to see who was watching as I stealthily made my way over the threshold. 'I've called in sick to the brewery,' he told me. His voice was strained but not hostile. 'Susie's in too much of a state to settle the baby.' I nodded but said nothing yet – I didn't know what the situation was. 'I wanted her to get her head down but she can't. Go through, Susie's in the kitchen,' he told me, opening the door to the small sitting room with the cramped scullery out the back. Mrs Bunyard was cleaning the already spotless worktops. 'She's gone through half a bottle of fairy liquid today,' her new husband whispered conspiratorially in my ear.

'Ah, Nurse,' Mrs Bunyard greeted me, pulling off her yellow rubber gloves. She was almost business-like despite still being in a peach full-length nightdress with angel sleeves, her hair loosely tied up with a white ribbon. 'It's all right, I've told him everything,' she confessed, clicking on the kettle and taking harvest-gold coffee mugs from the wrought-iron mug tree.

'It was a horrible place, Nurse,' continued Mrs Bunyard, her speech rapid and high-pitched. 'I had to sit there and listen to excuse after excuse from Charlie. How he wanted us to be a family when he got out – I said, "That's totally out of the question." When I told him I was married now and I'd given his baby away, he exploded,' she added, gripping the edges of the kitchen worktops with her palms as she rocked back and forth on her bare heels. 'The guards had to rush to hold him back and he shouted that his family would have the baby until I came to my senses. What about his rights? That we both belonged to him.' Mrs Bunyard bit the nail of her right finger, chipping the pearlescent polish. 'He got three years, you see, so he'll be out by next Easter. He kept shouting "My baby", "My wife", "How could you?"'

She popped the lid of a fresh jar of Nescafé instant coffee and poured the scalding water straight onto the grounds, stirring the black liquid around and around with a spoon until it rang. 'And all the way home I stared out the window of the car and I thought the same. "My baby", "How could I?", "How could I?" And as I was putting the key in the lock of our front door I knew something had changed – I had to get my Michelle back. Not because Charlie wants to have her, though God knows I don't want that, but because *I* want her. My baby, I want her back,' she finished, handing me the harvest-gold mug.

Alan Bunyard hovered in the doorway, the three of us still standing, unable to sit down. 'As soon as Aly got home I told him everything. He looked so hurt, Nurse. He didn't say anything at all for ages.'

'I wasn't angry, Nurse,' her husband interjected. 'I was upset she hadn't told me before,' he explained, never lifting his eyes from the linoleum kitchen floor. 'It was a lot to take in.'

'I was too scared to tell you before, Aly,' his wife cried out, rushing to touch his arm.

'I know, love. There'll be talk, but we can live with that, can't we?' he soothed.

Susan Bunyard nodded. She turned back to face me, her small hand in his, and announced, 'We want little Michelle to come and live with us, don't we, Aly?' Mr Bunyard nodded. I felt for Alan Bunyard – you could see the pain in his eyes. Susan Bunyard and I exchanged glances; we'd both thought he was only a village lad who drank too much, lived under the rule of his overbearing mother, and stumbled into marriage and fatherhood because he'd got her pregnant. We'd assumed he'd refuse to raise another man's child, possibly casting his new wife aside and leaving her to the likes of Charlie Carter.

We'd underestimated him.

'It's made me see things in a new light, Nurse,' Alan Bunyard added. 'Me, Susie and little Sharon – that's my family. I need to put them first. Not the lads I used to knock about with, not my relatives and certainly not my mother. Michelle, well, she's a part of Susie and Sharon. I can see it's breaking her heart. I've not exactly been a saint myself.'

Susan Bunyard reached up on tiptoes and kissed him on the cheek. 'Thank you,' she murmured. 'But we've got another problem. We rang my Aunty Mildred. We decided not to say we wanted Michelle to come and live with us, just that we'd like to visit her so she could meet baby Sharon. But she said no and hung up. We've tried to ring, and ring, but she's not picking up.'

'We'll drive over and demand to see Michelle,' Mr Bunyard suggested, his colour rising and a red hue spreading up his neck to the tips of his ears.

'I don't think that would help, Aly. We can't turn up, guns blazing. Michelle doesn't know who we are – I don't want to frighten her,' countered his wife. 'I don't want her first memory of me to be shouting the odds in the street.'

'I don't know what else we can do, love,' admitted her husband, putting his arm around her shoulder and pulling her close to him.

'Could you ring her, Nurse? Aunty Mildred might listen to you, a figure of authority, like.'

I gulped. 'The first step would be me telephoning the Welfare Department and getting a social worker assigned to your case. Saying that you've been denied access and we'd like to establish visits with a view to having the child back with her mother.'

'Would you do that for us?' asked Mrs Bunyard.

'Yes, of course. But it won't happen overnight and you'll need to be prepared to answer a lot of personal questions. If your aunty keeps on refusing it might mean going to court.'

'You mean a lot of busybody social workers poking their noses in?' Alan asked, a look of disgust creeping over his face.

Susan peeked up at him. 'Is it too much?' she asked in a small quivering voice.

He shook himself. 'If we must, we must,' he acquiesced.

Susan Bunyard gave a huge sigh of relief.

'Remember, it won't be the same process as when social services remove a child. Michelle isn't with your aunty because you did anything wrong, Mrs Bunyard. I can support you by saying you'll provide a loving and stable home. But it will take time and ultimately we have to do what's best for Michelle.'

'Surely it's best for Michelle to be with her mother,' barked Mr Bunyard.

'Calm down, Aly. The nurse is only explaining how it'll work. I can see it from Michelle's point of view. She doesn't know us, even if Aunty had said, "Yes, have her back," with the best will in the world we couldn't have rolled up there and brought her home, though God knows I want to.'

Mr Bunyard huffed. 'I suppose.'

'You're absolutely right, Mrs Bunyard. I'll go straight back to the office and call the Children's Department if you want me to.

Expect a letter and a visit in the next few weeks – we can at least get things moving.'

'Just think, Aly. Yesterday, I thought I'd never see Michelle again, that she'd never know me. Never know how much I longed for her. That I was the worst mother in the world. And now, if we hope and keep our cool, I could hold her again.'

# 12

It felt like the rest of October was a waiting game. The Bunyard family were never far from my thoughts. The quick telephone call to the Children's Department turned into hours as we got things rolling. When a social worker eventually returned my urgent request I was pleasantly surprised to discover it was Chris Jentry, whom I'd been out with on my student health visitor training the year before. We got chatting and I was so wrapped up in the Bunyards' affairs that my date with Nick that Friday evening completely slipped my mind. The result being he'd barely spoken to me since – and I couldn't really blame him. Of course he did his duty, announced the mothers' interest group, chatted about village matters when we bumped into each other, but that fragile fleeting intimacy of something more had evaporated.

I did what I was always did – threw myself into my work. We already had more than 20 mums coming to the Mothers' Interest Group, baby clinic was even more frantic now we had the bus service and there had been a rush of new arrivals, including Jackie Bowyer's waters breaking one morning at Mums and Toddlers to great excitement. But barely a thing had happened to get Mrs Bunyard any nearer to seeing her daughter. The only sign of progress being made were letters asking Dr Drake and me to write reports on the family. With her being new to the village the mediating doctor didn't know Susan, but he'd known Alan all his life. Fortunately, Dr Drake didn't drag his heels on submitting the paperwork, only requiring background from me and an appointment with the family. I was grateful it was Dr Drake and not his less capable partner. Dr Botten had become ever more tightly wound as the nights drew in. When I telephoned the surgery he had refused to come out to see Valerie Milstead's baby Michael, slurring his words and grumbling about better things to do before hanging up. I'd seen for myself there was mould on Miss Milstead's bedroom walls at Hollow Prospect, resulting in an increasingly bad chest for both her and the baby. I often thought back to a pair of babies who'd had to be put into steam tents at Hackney as a result of bronchitis from terrible living conditions – I hoped it wouldn't come to that.

It made my blood boil to see how comfortably her uncles lived while Valerie's life was like something out of *Tess of the d'Urbervilles*. Some weeks I had to go twice if her uncles were around; they did not take kindly to me calling. Her Uncle Ray in particular had come in during my last visit and mumbled a protest at my presence, 'Never mind all your gossiping, where's my dinner?' Then he looked at me leeringly: 'Who's she again?' he asked.

'She's the health visitor, Uncle Ray,' replied Valerie.

He shuffled out of the room, his grey-haired brother waiting for him in the doorway.

'Who's the busybody?' asked Uncle Donald.

'Authorities. Least said,' answered his aged brother.

It was already dark when I arrived at Mrs Wimble's on the last Monday of October. The air was misty and crisp, and late-autumn leaves created a carpet of coppers on the path through her corner of Fairy Woods, making a satisfying crunch beneath my feet as I approached the house. A wisp of smoke arose from the crooked chimney of Peasblossom. I'd taken to keeping a big stick propped up against an old Rowan tree on the other side of the fence to ward off Mrs Wimble's attacking gander. Fantasies of goose for Christmas dinner frequently filled my thoughts when I saw a flap of white feathers and heard that terrible honking sound. I braced myself for the onslaught but made my way to the kitchen door with a box of groceries surprisingly unmolested. Every week there seemed to be more and more cats – I must admit at times I wanted to put a peg on my nose.

The van driver from the village grocery had remarked to Mrs Wimble a fortnight ago that her home had '*le odeur de pisse le chat*' and had been barred from the property. Now I picked up her regular order from the shop on my way to see her and was visiting weekly rather than monthly. When I collected her supplies that morning, the grocer had remarked, 'Careful she doesn't put a hex on you, now, Nurse. That old place wants pulling down, gives me the creeps.' I didn't say anything. Standing in her kitchen there was some truth in the grocer's unkind words – 'health hazard' didn't come close to describing Mrs Wimble's insalubrious living conditions. I was at a loss to know where to unpack her provisions; she didn't have a fridge and every surface and cupboard was occupied by her feline companions or bunches of herbs and beakers. The elderly botanist continued to refuse point-blank to have the Welfare Department come in but I didn't know much longer she could go on like this. I thought I could hear voices coming from the sitting room.

'Hello, Mrs Wimble. I've got your groceries,' I called through.

Mrs Wimble shuffled into the kitchen, using a blackthorn stick as a cane, dressed in her usual multiple layers of onion-dyed woollens with her customary dressing gown as a coat and Wellington boots for slippers, a bunch of cow parsley in her hand.

'Do you have a visitor?' I asked.

'Certainly not,' she huffed.

I could have sworn I'd heard voices. 'What's that for, Mrs Wimble?' I enquired.

'Never you mind, Miss Hill.' She coughed badly, a persistent rattle on her chest. 'Did you bring my sugar?'

'Yes, it's all in here. Your cough sounds much worse. I could drive you into Totley and have Dr Drake examine you if you won't have him here.'

'I haven't been into Totley for 10 years,' she scolded me. 'I don't need that old quack poking about – he's as old as I am and completely gaga. I've got some rue that will do nicely, thank you.'

She gave me such a firm look that I dared not press further for fear she would rescind her invitation to let me visit. 'The gander didn't get me today. Have you put him in the pen?' I asked.

'No, the fox got him. Took his head clean off last night. It was a bloodbath of feathers and noise, quite macabre.'

'Oh, I'm sorry,' I sympathised, feeling guilty and relieved.

'That fox has been prowling around for months. My Gray gander was getting on, like everything else round here. Mr Fox bided his time until Gray was no match for his sharp jaws and got him in the end. I hope he made that damn fox a chewy meal,' she cursed, her steely grey eyes becoming moist and rheumy.

Mrs Wimble's world was becoming smaller and smaller. Her inaccessible ramshackle house confined her to the dilapidated kitchen, parlour and yard. The sofa in the sitting room was piled high with newspapers, brown woollen tights, charcoal cardigans and crimson cushions with large holes that I suspected mice were squatting in. Pairs of dingy grey knickers were drying on a clothes horse in front of the fire and chipped plates of half-eaten meals littered the floor. The balls and balls of wool and knitting needles had been shoved into a wicker basket and left in the corner. I started to pick up a few things but Mrs Wimble flopped into her great armchair snapping, 'Don't fuss.'

'Where are you sleeping now?' I asked. Mrs Wimble pointed her stick in the direction of the battered sofa. 'That will only make your chest worse.'

'I can't manage the stairs,' she informed me gruffly.

'We could arrange for a nice clean comfortable bed to be brought into here,' I suggested, but she quickly cut me off.

'No, no, no. No more of that, Miss Hill, or we shall fall out,' Mrs Wimble told me.

'All right. But would you consider letting Nurse Bates call?'

'Who?'

'The district nurse,' I prompted.

'That flighty blonde.'

I ignored that. 'Nurse Bates is very kind and discreet. I think if you let her pop in to do a little bit of care as well as my visits, you'd have a better week.'

Mrs Wimble closed her eyes and pressed her lips tightly together and sighed deeply. 'Once a week, on a trial basis.'

I agreed though we both knew this situation couldn't continue for much longer but I was glad to give Laura Bates the all-clear to call.

Feeling quite swish in my new dark-brown knee-high boots and three-quarter-length camel leather coat I sauntered along to the Village Hall for my first professionals' quarterly meeting arm in arm with Hermione, who'd shared an early supper with me at Ivy Cottage. My colleague looked like Ava Gardner in her skirted mahogany velvety coat with broad leopard-print lapels, a smart deep chestnut-coloured fedora tilted roguishly on her shiny dark head. We passed some children from the village school pushing a guy on a cart made from a crate and old pram wheels. 'Penny for the guy,' they called to us. Hermione immediately reached into her purse and gave them a few coins. I recognised one of the children as Neil Bowyer.

'How's your mum getting on with the new baby, Neil?' I asked, handing over some money.

'I don't know why she needed another one. It cries and then Stacy cries, it's driving me round the bend,' he replied, before wheeling the guy off down the Totley Main Road.

'Well, you did ask,' Hermione said, laughing. 'How many does Mrs Bowyer have now, three?'

'Four, there's Jenny too. All in the little two-bed flat over Totley Garage. I can see from Neil's point of view it's not much fun right now.'

'Is "it" a boy or a girl?'

'A boy, Gordon. I haven't seen him yet, they're still under Nurse Higgins's care.'

'Are you excited for your first professionals' meeting?'

'I'm very thrilled Dr Mia Kellmer Pringle is the speaker. I've read her book and I watched her on *Controversy* on BBC2 last night,' I enthused as we reached the door of the Village Hall.

'Ah yes, *Why Young Children Need Full-Time Mothers* – it's certainly a controversial point of view, Sarah,' Hermione remarked with a raised perfectly pencilled eyebrow. 'And one I don't wholeheartedly agree with; I can see work provides families with economic assistance and social benefits for the mother. For some being at home with children is a joy, while for others it can be a depressing drudge. Each family has their own needs.'

The hall was already buzzing. I spied Mrs King pouring sherries and Flo going around with a tray, doling out cheese on crackers. Nitty Nora had our manager Miss Presnell pinned in a corner, pouring poison into her ear, no doubt. Nick Shepherd saw me, gave an aloof smile and then turned his back on me, intent on examining a few old black and white photos on the wall he must have seen a hundred times before. It smarted a little. At the centre of the room Nurse Higgins looked incredible in an emerald-green jumpsuit with wide flares skimming a pair of white leather sandals. She was deep in conversation with a slim woman in a wide-brimmed mustard hat, a herringbone suit and beige silk blouse. I recognised her at once from her television appearance: it was Dr Mia Kellmer Pringle.

Hermione went to assist Mrs King with the drinks, assuring me they didn't need my help and encouraging me to get to know the array of community professionals gathered together. Laura Bates gave me a painful smile from across the room. She'd taken her place on the first row of chairs in front of the stage. A young policeman was sitting next to her talking very ardently, his thigh pressing into hers, his hand kept straying onto her knee. She'd crossed her legs to knock him off but completely undeterred he continued the conversation and put his hand back on her knee again. I marched over.

'Nurse Bates, sorry to talk shop but I wondered if you'd had the chance to visit Peasblossom yet?' I unceremoniously interrupted.

'Oh yes, I wanted to talk to you about that,' cried Laura, jumping up and dislodging her unwanted admirer.

'Thanks for rescuing me from Constable Octopus, Sarah,' Laura whispered as we scurried away.

'You're welcome. What a total creep!'

'I did want to talk to you about Mrs Wimble, though. I went a little after four o'clock this afternoon to give her a wash and brush up.'

'Did she not let you in? She promised,' I grumbled.

'No, I managed to get in there now that flaming goose is gone. It was when I arrived, I could have sworn she was talking to someone.'

'I thought that yesterday. But she said there was no one else in the house and there wasn't sight nor sound of another soul.'

'Yes, same here. But truly, I did hear another voice. And she was waffling on about gardening, or herbs or something,' continued the district nurse.

'She and her husband were both botanists.'

'Oh goodness,' exclaimed Laura grasping my arm. 'You don't think it's his ghost, do you?'

'Don't be a goose yourself,' I teased. 'I talk to myself sometimes. Don't you? It's part of living alone.'

'The odd word perhaps,' admitted Laura. 'But not whole conversations. It gives me the heebie-jeebies.'

Miss Presnell called us to order and we took our seats away from the eager young policeman on the second row. Chris Jentry sat down on my left.

'It's lovely to see you again,' the social worker greeted me, leaning over to kiss me on the cheek. He was in his early forties, with shoulder-length sandy hair that was greying at the temples. He was wearing the same zip-up dark-green cardigan and fraying brown corduroy trousers he'd worn practically every day of my week of training with him last year. 'We must go for a cuppa sometime to catch up. You were such an eager student I'd love to hear how you're getting on.'

I heard a loud snort from behind me. I turned and there was Nick. All broody and smouldering in a pristine suede zip-up cardigan in a diamond print.

'Hi,' he said smoothly.

'Hi,' I replied quietly before quickly turning to face the front, keeping my eyes firmly fixed on the stage.

The Viennese psychologist began, 'If children are to enjoy their lives, develop their full potential and grow into participating, contributing adults within our society it is necessary their physical, emotional, social and intellectual needs are met. At present for many children their physical needs are met but there is more that can be done by parents and professionals like you to ensure a holistic approach is taken to nurture their psycho-social needs.'

'I need another sherry, if the whole talk is going to be like this,' muttered Laura.

I shushed her and felt cross I'd missed a bit. Then tuned back in to Dr Kellmer Pringle. 'Experiences and opportunities in the early years of life greatly influence later development. Human capacity to learn is such the newborn child can adapt to widely different environments. Genetics are the raw material but it is experience and environment that truly shape most of us.'

'Oh, yawn. This is like having to listen to my dad,' grumbled Laura.

'Is he a psychologist?'

'No, a doctor in Hernia Bay.'

'Where?' I asked.

'It's what I like to call Herne Bay on account of my dad's patients,' giggled Laura.

'Emotional development is not the same as IQ. This is based on educational testing and only serves to measure a person's ability to perform well on tasks similar to the tests. It has led to the false impression that doing well in tests necessarily means a greater competence in coping, later on, with life in general – it does not where intellect has been nurtured over psycho-social development,' Dr Kellmer Pringle told us.

'Actually, I'll remember that next time my dad starts going on about my O-levels,' perked up Laura. 'I may not have an A in Biology, Father, but I'm a dab hand with an old dear needing the commode.'

'Laura!' I scolded. Dr Kellmer Pringle wasn't the most charismatic of speakers but I found her research fascinating.

'Newborn baby, toddler, pre-schooler, child, adolescent and every person in this room share the same emotional needs which must be nourished throughout our lives if we are to become not only valued members of society but also to value ourselves – if we are to be happy with who we are,' explained the psychologist.

I thought about my mother and her daily struggles with five young children. The middle child in me felt a lump in my throat. 'What about me? Was I happy?' I pondered.

'It is the early years that are the most sensitive period for our emotional development – more progress, change and development take place in the first years of life than at any other time. The brain itself undergoes the most rapid growth in the first two years, and young children are most susceptible to wide experiences, stimulation or in some cases isolation that have lasting and irreversible effects – therefore we might have no conscious memory of life as babies but what we learn about ourselves and the world around us, good or bad, is lasting and irreversible. In my book *The Needs of Children*, which some of you may have read, I identify the need for love and security, the need for new experiences, the need for praise and recognition, and the need for responsibility,' asserted Dr Kellmer Pringle.

'Heavy stuff,' Laura hissed in my ear but I was hooked.

'Some of you may have seen me on BBC2 last night.' There were nods around the room. 'Not every child can have a full-time mother. Not every child has a mother and there are parents as we sadly know who are incapable of meeting their child's needs. But social scientists continue to ignore the concept of "mother-love" regarding it as unmeasurable, sentimental or both. Maybe you as professionals have undervalued it? Motherly love in infancy and childhood is as important for mental health as are vitamins and proteins for physical health. We might call this attachment.

Attachment to the person who is the main carer for a child, which in most families today is their mother is everything.'

'I think she's wonderful,' I whispered to Laura.

'You would,' she teased.

This was the missing piece for me. Families didn't just need answers to physical problems but emotional support for the whole family. I didn't think mothers had to be full-time in every family – it was too sweeping – but whoever was caring for a child could put their emotional needs at the centre of their care, couldn't they? A happy baby needs a happy family. It got me thinking about how to meet the emotional needs of children, mums and dads, which I still think about now. Dear reader, in that moment I saw the type of health visitor I wanted to be.

# 13

'Have you ever had a family with a poltergeist?' I asked my colleagues over tea and one of Mrs King's delicious homemade Maids of Honour.

'Now that's a question,' said Mrs King with a laugh.

'People are always thinking their babies are chatting to ghosts – it's baby babble,' Hermione informed me.

'What do you know about The Old Watermill?' I tried a different tack.

'The Underdowns' place? They haven't been there long,' recollected Hermione. 'Less than a year as I recall. Didn't they buy it from the Hollemans, Beatie?'

'Yes, and the Hollemans had been there for centuries,' continued Mrs King.

'Centuries?' I asked.

'Oh yes, dear. The mill is seventeenth-century. Jack would know more about it,' said Mrs King.

Her husband was a master at the prep school in Malling.

'Why do you ask, Sarah? Not suddenly a local history buff, are you?' teased Hermione, giving me a quizzical stare over the nose of her tortoise-shell spectacles.

'Well, yesterday, at Mums and Toddlers I couldn't help but notice Mrs Underdown wasn't herself. She's usually so vibrant and very good at leading the singing. But she kept getting all the words mixed up, like her mind was wandering. And afterwards she could barely keep her eyes open. She looked not just tired, more at the end of her tether.'

'Yes, I've noticed the poor girl's looking a bit peaky when I've seen her about the village,' sympathised Mrs King.

'Dean, her little boy, looked tired too. He's usually running around creating havoc but yesterday he curled up on one of the playmats and had a nap,' I told them.

'Wasn't he the little card who got his head stuck in a saucepan a few weeks ago?' Hermione remembered.

'Yes, that's him. But yesterday he was like a little shadow of his former self and he's a very sweet child. I popped to the loo and found Mrs Underdown in a bad way. She was white as a sheet and shaking. She told me she'd been sick and was getting hardly any sleep. Dean keeps waking them up in the night but until a few weeks ago he'd been a good sleeper. She and her husband are wiped out.'

'Oh dear. Are you going to give them some advice on sleep?' enquired Hermione.

'I asked her if she'd like me to pop round to talk about bedtime routines. She said yes, it was getting difficult to get Dean to go to bed, and he wasn't sleeping through. But none of them were, because the ghost keeps waking them up,' I finished.

'What ghost?' asked my surprised colleagues.

'She got a bit embarrassed and cagey. Started apologising that I must think she was barmy and in no state to take care of Dean. I tried to reassure her that wasn't the case. We agreed I'd see them this afternoon at home. But I've no idea what to expect. I'm a nurse, not an exorcist,' I added, trying to add some humour to my tale, but I felt completely out of my depth.

'Proceed with caution, Miss Hill,' advised Mrs King. 'There are rumours about The Old Watermill and the Hollemans.' She shook her head, 'But it was no more than village gossip.' She bit her lip, considering my predicament. 'Fear is a very powerful emotion, so be careful, Sarah.'

'Sarah, just to warn you. Mrs Underdown's husband is a good 20 years older than her,' Hermione told me.

'Thanks for the warning,' I said.

'And don't forget, it's Halloween tomorrow,' Hermione added with a mischievous smile. 'You might want to get your besom broom out.'

I parked my green Mini in front of the octagon-shaped white weather-boarded Old Watermill. At three storeys high it cast a long chilly shadow over me. I looked up at the mill's motionless sails and fantail and felt uneasy. I'd never had a case like this before, I didn't know what to expect. Should I go in with an open mind? Was this situation a fantasy, illness or simply attention seeking? What were the implications for Dean? What was worse; living in a house with a genuine poltergeist or having parents who were delusional? Why shouldn't it be a ghost? What was going on with Mrs Underdown? I'd always found her a really pleasant sensible woman, so why would she make something like this up? I needed to put all questions out of my head – listen, Sarah, listen, I instructed myself. Taking a few deep breaths and wishing I'd done a few of Dr Drake's meditative breathing exercises before setting out, I attempted to calm myself before knocking on the door of the mill. It was opened by a man of about 50 in a blue-denim suit with thick wavy blonde-grey hair. I remembered Hermione's warning about Mrs Underdown's husband being much older.

'Hello, Mr Underdown. I'm Sarah Hill, the health visitor. Your wife asked me to call this afternoon.'

'Hello, Nurse, we've been expecting you. Come in,' he replied with a wry smile. 'Yvonne, the nurse is here,' he called.

I heard footsteps running down the spiral staircase of the mill before Mrs Underdown appeared in a dark-pink matching shirt and skirt. She was barefoot and as usual her thick blonde curls were kept in place by a matching headscarf. It was unusual for her to be wearing wide white-framed sunglasses indoors in late autumn, but I guessed this was to hide the huge dark circles under her eyes. She'd applied powder and glossy peach lipstick but you could still see how pale she was underneath it all.

'Thanks for coming, Nurse,' she greeted me. 'I've managed to put Dean down for a nap after lunch,' she told me. 'Not that any of us could eat much.'

'The sleep will do him good,' I said.

'Yes. God knows he needs it.'

The man followed me looking very amused – I didn't think his wife's distress was very funny. The mill sitting room was octagonal with exposed brickwork and windows on four sides. A large, sparsely decorated dresser stood before the passageway to the kitchen. Miss Elena Moon was seated in a chintz armchair in front of a log-burner fireplace; I recalled she was Mrs Underdown's aunt. Opposite Miss Moon was a man wearing a blue and white plaid double-knit suit and navy polo-neck jumper, who also had blonde-grey wavy hair.

'What do you look so tickled about?' Mrs Underdown asked the man who'd opened the door.

'The nurse thought I was your husband,' he said, chuckling.

'Oh, Dad! Why didn't you say something?' Mrs Underdown scolded.

'Hardly,' called out the man in the plaid suit, getting up from his chair. 'You're a bit long in the tooth for a young family, aren't you, Abe?' Mr Underdown chided his father-in-law as he stroked his hair back into place with a little comb, but actually the two men were like two peas in a pod.

'Hush now, Eli,' Mrs Underdown told her husband. 'You're as bad as each other. I don't want the nurse to think this is all a joke. Sit down, would you, Nurse?' she invited.

'I'll get some coffee on,' said Miss Moon. I felt for her as she walked unsteadily down the passage to the kitchen, pausing momentarily by the dresser for support and sighing deeply.

'She's very sensitive to the vibrations,' Mr Moon divulged in a conspiratorial whisper.

'Dean is having scary dreams about monsters and it's getting difficult to get him to sleep,' began Mrs Underdown. 'I've started sitting at the top of the stairs waiting for him to drop off. I usually put on his night light and read him a story, and then I kiss him goodnight and go, and he's out like a light. But lately I can hear him chatting to someone – keeping himself awake. At first I thought it was nothing but in the last few weeks other things have started happening too.' She paused.

'What sort of things, Mrs Underdown?'

'You won't believe me, Nurse. I scarcely believe myself. But at midnight as that long clock over there chimes and we're all in bed, the house starts to quiver. I've lost so many ornaments off the mantelpiece and cups and plates off the dresser in the last few weeks. When we run downstairs to see what's happening the lights flash on and off. We're terrified. It's been like that every night except Sundays. It's never happened on a Sunday, has it, Eli?

Mr Underdown's smug grin had been replaced with a grey look. He patted his wife's knee reassuringly. 'I asked Dean who he was talking to. He said it was a soldier,' he added.

'A soldier? Like GI Joe in green combats?' I asked.

'That's what I thought,' said Mrs Underdown. 'He got one of those dolls for his third birthday. Eli bought it him and I thought it was a bit soon for playing war games – he's still a baby.'

'It's a toy, Yvonne. You don't want him to grow up to be a sissy, do you?' her husband chipped in.

'Anyway,' continued Mrs Underdown, shaking out her glossy curls with a touch of defiance, 'he said his soldier looked like Captain Hook, with long curly hair and a sword and a big black hat with a feather in it and long boots.'

'Something he's seen in a storybook perhaps?' I suggested.

'Yes, Nurse. I'd agree with you if it wasn't for the goings-on at midnight. It's frightening Dean. It's scaring the hell out of me. And you, Eli, you can't explain it either. And when you don't get enough sleep you can't see things clearly – I don't want to think.'

Mr Underdown shook his head and looked at his hands. 'There are stories too, Nurse, about The Old Watermill,' explained her husband. 'I'm not from Totley. Yvonne and I were living in Maidstone but she wanted to be near her family. When the Hollemans sold the land for the new housing estate, The Old Watermill came on the market and it seemed like a good opportunity, only now I'm not so sure.'

'What stories?' I asked, taking a cup from Aunty Elena when she returned with the coffee.

'I don't believe them. Village nonsense,' Eli Underdown dismissed.

'Dad, would you tell the nurse?' asked Yvonne.

Abe Moon leant forward in his seat, savouring the moment. 'When Elena and I were knee-high our grandfather used to tell us how Totley had been a supporter of the Cavaliers in the Civil War. Oliver Cromwell's men had pursued Cavaliers from Totley Grange into the village. An earl's youngest son, a soldier, hid in this mill. When the Roundheads discovered him, they executed him and tied him to one of the sails as a warning to other Royalists. It's his spirit that cannot rest, od rabbit it! People say the

Hollemans gave him shelter and he's all put out now they've left,' finished Mr Moon with a flourish.

We were all speechless; I didn't know what to suggest. Four pairs of eyes were on me waiting for a solution. I gulped and was saved by Dean's cries as he woke up from his nap.

'He's only had 15 minutes,' despaired Mrs Underdown as she ran off to see to her son.

'It's more than monsters under the bed, Nurse,' Abe Moon told me. 'It's a poltergeist and I don't think that's covered by the NHS,' he added with a wink as Mrs Underdown returned with Dean in her arms. Bless the little lad, he hadn't had his sleep out and was clutching a fistful of his mother's hair in his small chubby hand. The child was pink-cheeked and had beads of sweat on his brow. Yvonne rocked Dean back and forth until he fell back asleep on her and they settled together on the sofa.

'While you've got the opportunity, why don't you try and get some sleep yourself, Mrs Underdown?' I suggested.

'What a good idea,' agreed Aunty Elena. She immediately fetched a rug and tucked in her niece and great nephew.

'What do you say, Nurse? This business has got our Yvonne all fanteeg. Do you think it's wrongtaking or there's something in Dean's soldier?' probed Abe Moon.

I was undecided and played for time. 'Would you mind if I had a look around before I left?'

'Help yourself, Nurse,' answered Mr Underdown.

'Have you spoken to the vicar about this?' I enquired.

'Father Nick?' replied Miss Moon in a worried, timid voice. 'Oh, no. He'd think we were Satanists. What would the rest of the village say?'

'I'm sure he wouldn't think anything like that. We'd both keep it confidential. But Reverend Shepherd might be able to help. Maybe come and bless the house,' I proposed.

'Would you ask him, Nurse?' requested Mrs Underdown as her eyes started to close.

Nick was barely talking to me at the moment. I didn't know if he would help with something like this. I couldn't imagine him being very receptive. 'Perhaps it would be better if …'

'Please,' begged Miss Moon. 'He'll take it more seriously from you. He'll think we're a bunch of loonies.'

'If you like,' I acquiesced.

Mr Moon showed me out as his family tried to rest. 'Now's the time to get it done, Nurse,' he advised. 'It'll be finger-cold from tonight and tomorrow's Halloween. Now don't tell me that's just coincidence. We have an obligation to put this right,' he informed me, all humour now gone from his voice.

Before I left the mill I walked around the garden to get a better look at the place. Looking up at those sails I couldn't help but shudder. The garden backed onto a field filled with oil-seed rape. It looked so beautiful lit up by the dipping afternoon sun creating a hazy cloud of bronze and gold. I felt drawn to it and walked into the field to gather my thoughts. In the distance I could see Totley Grange high on the hill behind the new Watermill Estate. Those Cavaliers must have run this way trying to escape, I deduced. The field was dappled by grey smudges amongst the crops. As I walked along the perimeter I realised those smudges were the bodies of wood pigeons lying dead around the boundaries of the house. I had to go and see Nick.

I returned to the clinic to telephone Nick. I'd never set foot in The Parsonage and didn't feel I could just turn up. Laura Bates was sitting at my desk, enjoying a piece of Mrs King's homemade shortbread.

'Making yourself at home?' I teased.

'I'm been waiting for you an age,' she informed me with a

mouth full, scattering crumbs on my desk. 'It's about Mrs Wimble. I'll go and see her again tomorrow. If she's giving gardening tips to souls from beyond the grave we'll have to call the Welfare Department, or a priest or something.'

'Oh no, not you as well!' I complained.

'What's the matter?' Laura asked with a bruised look.

'Sorry. Shall we go together on Monday morning? I think I'll be tied up tomorrow.'

'Yes, that's fine by me. Safety in numbers and I don't fancy investigating phantom horticulturists on All Hallows' Eve,' she said with a chuckle. 'Well, I've got a bit more scrubbing to do before the day is out. Thank Mrs King for the shortbread for me,' she added as she jumped up. 'I will meet you in Fairy Woods on Monday and make sure you wear a crucifix or something,' joked the district nurse, pulling her cape up over her face like Count Dracula as she departed backwards through the door letting it bang shut. Laura was in good humour but I felt all of a quiver. What was it with all the spooky goings-on in Totley at the moment? I rang Nick.

'Hello, The Parsonage, Totley,' he answered.

'It's Sarah Hill.'

'Long time, no see.'

'I wanted to ask if you'd help me with one of your parishioners.'

'You'd better come up to The Parsonage then, if it's not too much trouble?'

'Thank you. When would be a good time?'

'No time like the present. I'll see you in 10 minutes,' he instructed and hung up.

Ten minutes later I was in Nick's very comfortable parsonage. I had popped into Ivy Cottage for a few minutes before to brush my hair and put on some lipstick. The Parsonage had a good view over the whole of Totley, with its sloping garden connected to both the churchyard and road. Yet it was still private, surrounded by a neat high laurel hedge. Nick was waiting for me at the door and watched me open the front gate and walk down the garden path to meet him.

He smiled. 'Welcome to my humble abode. Can I get you some tea?'

I looked about the parlour while Nick was busy in the kitchen, having shooed his housekeeper out the back door. It was a neat, comfortable room and a very large house for one person to rattle around in.

'I'm glad you came,' he told me.

'Are you?'

'Yes, that you still feel we can work together for the sake of the community.'

Reverend Shepherd listened without comment or censure as I told him about the Underdowns, the soldier, the stories about The Old Watermill, the lights flashing and the smashed crockery.

'Do you believe in God?' he asked me.

'Yes, I do,' I replied.

'And the Underdowns?'

'I believe so.'

'There's a reason we renounce the devil in baptism, Sarah. Why we pray for deliverance from evil in the Lord's Prayer.'

'More things in heaven and earth,' I commented.

'Exactly. We pray for protection. I can minister to the Underdowns if they wish but I can't do much more.'

'Could you bless the house at least?'

He pondered for a moment. 'It's not that, I'm afraid. I don't have any experience in this sort of thing. I don't have the proper insurance.' I stifled a laugh. 'It's not funny, Sarah. Deliverance can only be exercised by a priest authorised by the diocesan bishop.'

'Mr Bourne's father?'

He looked surprised. 'You know him?'

'Of him. I saw him and Miss Bourne at the Harvest Festival service.'

'Oh yes, of course. As I said, I can minister to them but I need someone to accompany me. The Church has guidelines on this sort of thing.'

'Does it?' I was surprised.

'Oh yes. It's advised I have a health professional with me in case anyone gets hurt or if it turns out it isn't a spirit but the Underdowns' mental health that needs ministering too.'

'That sounds sensible.'

'You'll come with me?'

'Me?' I gasped.

'I can't think of anyone more appropriate.' I gulped and nodded in agreement. 'I'll need a little time to prepare. Shall we say tomorrow night?'

'Tomorrow?'

'Yes, is there a problem? You did come to me.'

'But it's 31 October tomorrow.'

'Oh Sarah, you aren't scared of children dressed up in old sheets, are you?' he said with a smirk.

I wasn't having Nick thinking I was a scaredy-cat. 'That's not a problem. When do you need me?'

'If we pray with Dean before bedtime. And then wait around until midnight and see what occurs.'

'Seven o'clock, then?'

He nodded. 'Can I leave it you to tell the Underdowns?' he requested, rising to his feet.

'Certainly.'

'Well, then, I shall meet you at The Old Watermill tomorrow at seven,' he told me.

Our interview was over.

\* \* \*

Dean must have wondered why his bedroom was so crowded that night. His mother and I watched from the doorway as the Reverend Shepherd knelt by his bed and prayed:

May the cross of the Son of God,
which is mightier than all the hosts of Satan
and more glorious than all the hosts of heaven,
abide with you in your going out and in your coming in.
By day and by night, at morning and at evening,
at all times and in all places may it protect and defend you.
From the wrath of evildoers, from the assaults of evil spirits,
from foes visible and invisible, from the snares of the devil,
from all passions that beguile the soul and body:
may it guard, protect and deliver you.
Amen.

Mr Underdown, Mr and Miss Moon were hovering on the spiral staircase behind us. We all of us bowed our heads, said 'Amen' and waited. Nothing happened. I don't know what we were expecting. The parson rose to his feet calmly and made the sign of the cross on Dean's forehead.

'May the peace of the Lord be with you and remain with you always, Amen.'

'Amen,' we all repeated once more in reverential hushed tones.

'Shall we let Mrs Underdown read Dean his bedtime story?' suggested Nick cheerfully.

'Sweet dreams,' I said to Dean. Wishing it would be true.

Mrs Underdown began reading *Peter Rabbit* in a small strained voice and we closed the door on mother and child.

'More tea, Vicar?' asked Abe Moon.

Nick smiled indulgently. 'I think Miss Hill and I will leave you in peace to continue your evening. Please go to bed as usual. We'll come back in a few hours and set up camp in the garden for a while and then if you would leave the back door open we'll come into the house just before midnight to see what occurs.'

Nick and I went on to The Good Intent. Ted the landlord had popped in plastic white fangs, slicked back his dark hair and put on a black cape with red lining. Totley's answer to Count Dracula was serving up Mill Farm Cider in skull-shaped cups.

'Can I tempt you, Nurse?' Ted asked with a twinkle.

'I'd have thought you were a bit old for this lark, Ted,' chided Nick.

'Just a bit of fun, Vicar,' conciliated the pub landlord. 'Can I tempt you to a cider-skull cup?'

'Pint of Totley Beer, if you please. Sarah?'

'I'll give a cider-skull cup a whirl,' I answered. Nick rolled his eyes and paid for the drinks.

'I'll expect to see you joining in with apple bobbing later, Nurse,' called Ted as we escaped his clutches in a quiet corner.

'I don't think so,' sneered the vicar.

'Oh, it sounds like fun,' I teased.

Nick took a long sip of his beer. I felt a bit silly now drinking out of a plastic skull. It was good cider but given the circumstances maybe a vodka and lime would have been more suitable. I decided to switch to ginger beer for the rest of the evening.

'We're finally on our date,' remarked Nick.

He'd caught me by surprise. Is that what this was? Hardly! 'I have apologised for that. For a Man of God you certainly hold a grudge,' I chastised. He looked bruised. We sat in silence for a while. The cider warmed me and I started to feel a little more relaxed. I leaned in and confided, 'I saw a ghost once.'

Nick looked at me curiously, his lip curling into a wry smile. 'Did you?'

'Yes, when I was about 13. I was coming home from a Halloween party at the village hall in Connel ...'

'Connel?'

'Near Oban, in Scotland.'

'Are you from Scotland?'

'We lived there for several years while my father led the building of the hydroelectric power station at Ben Cruachan.'

'Your father's a civil engineer?

'Yes.'

'I didn't know that. What's his name?'

'Eric Hill. Anyway,' I continued, 'we'd been ducking for apples and eating marshmallows on a string and I was walking home alone. I didn't know where my brother and sisters were ...'

'You've got siblings?' he interrupted again.

'Yes, two brothers and two sisters.'

'What are their names?'

Oh really, for heaven's sake. 'William, Jane, Bridget and Stephen,' I rattled off.

'Are you younger or older?'

'I'm in the middle.'

'That explains a lot.'

'Do you not want to hear my story? You're rather ruining it.'

'Sorry.'

I frowned and folded my arms. I wasn't going to say another word.

'I don't know very much about you, Sarah.'

I suppose that was true. I didn't know much about him either. What was our relationship? A few brief awkward exchanges in shops, halls and churchyards, a couple of telephone calls. A wave at the mothers' interest group. The only times we'd been alone were the night of the drunken kiss in the doorway of Ivy Cottage and yesterday in The Parsonage, in that neat, comfortable parlour.

There was no relationship. There was nothing between us really. Just a lot of hot and cold air.

'Life is more exciting when I'm with you. Less predictable. Please tell me your story,' he entreated.

'I was walking on my own through the village in the dark. I saw this shadowy figure drift out of the kirk and go into the churchyard. It was a man in a black fedora and long black coat. He cast a huge shadow onto the wall of the kirk but he didn't walk, he floated! He floated right into the churchyard and then he evaporated.'

'And you think that was a ghost?'

'Yes, I do.'

'And what do you think about Dean's soldier?'

'I don't know what to think.'

'Well, Ted's getting ready for the apple bobbing. Shall we finish our drinks and make a dash for it?'

'Good idea.'

A slither of a waning crescent moon lit up the street as we left the pub. It was a frosty sparkling evening. Hoar frost glistened on the bare trees and hedges as we followed the path down the hill back to The Old Watermill. It was like being wrapped in a cloak of midnight blue velvet. Before I realised he'd done it, Nick was holding my hand, his long elegant fingers entwined with mine. Miss Moon brought us a stack of rugs and delicious hot chocolate to keep out the cold. We made camp in the garden seated at a white wrought-iron table with matching chairs. Basking in the moonlight, we revelled in the bright stars so clear and brilliant in the country night sky. We watched as each of the lights went out on the small windows of the mill, knowing the family were tucked up in bed. Only the night light in Dean's window gave any illumination. We almost forgot why we were there until the stillness of the night was interrupted by Dean's cries and the lights went on. All the hairs on the back of my neck stood on end.

'Should we go in?' asked Nick.

'Give it a minute.'

We strained to hear what was happening through the darkness. The crying stopped and a couple of minutes later the lights went off once more.

'Just a nightmare,' I explained.

We waited and waited. There was nothing. I started to wonder if it was some elaborate Halloween prank. At 10 to midnight we went into the mill to wait upon Mrs Underdown's poltergeist. I sat with Nick in the sitting room. All the family were in bed. The long clock began to strike 12 and then the floor started to tremble and within seconds the whole house was shaking. Nick prayed once more:

Lord, we pray, this place
and drive far from it all the snares of the enemy.
Let your holy angels dwell here to keep us in peace,
and may your blessing be upon it evermore;
through Jesus Christ our Lord.
Amen.

But I couldn't focus. All about us everything was moving. Cups and saucers came off the dresser and smashed on the floor. The lights did flash and there was a blinding light in the window for a couple of seconds. The noise built to a roar that lasted only a moment and then faded away into a distant echo of sound and movement, leaving only the thud of feet from above us as the family rose from their beds. Mrs Underdown went straight to Dean's bedroom; the poor child was shrieking in fear with all the commotion. Mr Underdown ran down the spiral staircase to us in only his striped pyjamas, his hair sticking up at all angles revealing a bald patch.

'Did you see anything?' he cried out desperately.

'Not really,' I answered.

'I did. Come on,' said Nick, grabbing my hand. Without justification we ran out into the darkness. 'Did you see the light?'

In the distance I could see faint beams of light beyond the field where I'd found all those dead wood pigeons yesterday. I didn't want to go in there but before I could protest we were running along the track through the field. My heart was racing; I felt sick. I wanted to go back, but Nick had a tight hold of my hand.

'Nick, I want to check on Dean,' I called out, trying to pull away. The child was my priority, not ghost hunting.

But he kept a tight hold of my hand and shouted, 'Come on,' like a man possessed.

Breathlessly we came to the small clearing where they were building the Watermill Estate.

'There's your ghost,' cried Nick triumphantly.

The building site was aglow with the headlights of juggernauts loaded with building materials.

'What do you think you're doing?' Nick shouted angrily at the workmen. 'You're not supposed to come through the village at all. I'll be taking this up with the developer. Come on, Sarah. Let's explain to the Underdowns what's been making the house shake.'

We walked back through the fields hand in hand.

'So, it was the lorries coming through at midnight that was causing the mill to shake?'

'Yes, it must have been.'

'And the dead pigeons?'

'Farmers shoot them to stop them eating the crops.'

'And Dean's soldier?'

'Imagination.'

'That's not much of an explanation.'

'Let's see if it puts Mrs Underdown's mind to rest. If it does, that's good enough for me. Ghost or not, it's never harmed anyone. The family weren't upset by the ghost; it was the bumps in the night. And tomorrow morning I intend to put a stop to those once and for all.'

The Underdowns were mightily relieved and we all laughed over cocoa in the small hours before making our way home.

There was no more haunting at The Old Watermill. With undisturbed nights everything very quickly went back to normal. Dean did tell me once that he sometimes still saw his soldier but whether that was just his imagination or not I simply don't know.

Laura Bates and I decided to go undercover to get to the bottom of Mrs Wimble's mystery voices. At 10 o'clock on Monday morning we covertly parked at the bottom of the lane in Fairy Woods and crept down the path to Peasblossom, hoping to arrive incognito. We peeked through the windows into Mrs Wimble's sitting room. Cats on the prowl were clearly the kings of this domain as well as the kitchen. Two huge moggies slept on either end of the mantelpiece like ornaments, kittens mewling from open drawers in the sideboard. I could smell it through the window. As we'd suspected the elderly botanist was indeed talking to someone; through the thin pane of glass we could hear her muttering.

'We'll not starve. There's oyster mushrooms and winter chanterelles nearby that will make a delicious salad.'

To our astonishment we heard a man's voice say. 'Gorse is great in salads.'

'No, I've told you gorse is on the moorlands – there's none in Fairy Woods, you silly man,' carped Mrs Wimble. 'You'll have to like it or lump it.' She started to cough and wheeze.

The man's voice then continued. 'I am partial to chickweed soup.'

'I'll give you that,' she responded in a conciliatory tone. 'Though, I don't think my back and knees are up to picking chickweed this winter,' she added sorrowfully, lifting up her leg. It was bruised black and blue.

'Who is she talking to?' whispered Laura.

I shrugged my shoulders. 'We'd better go in and get to the bottom of this.'

We knocked on the door of the cottage. As usual she didn't bother to reply so we went in.

'Mrs Wimble,' I called. 'It's Sarah Hill. I'm here with Laura Bates, the district nurse.'

'Come in, girls,' replied Mrs Wimble. She was standing alone in the sitting room, dressed in a pair of men's pyjamas and smoking a pipe. 'My late husband's,' she replied coquettishly, giving us a twirl. 'Have you met Derek? He knows rather a lot about wildlife, though his knowledge of flora and fauna in our native Kent leaves a lot to be desired.'

We looked about us perplexed – there was no one else in the room. Then we heard the man's voice again. 'From winter foraging, we move onto how some plants actually discourage pollinating insects.' It was coming from the radio.

'He does go on a bit, I'm afraid,' she whispered. 'And he doesn't listen very well at all,' Mrs Wimble remarked on the radio presenter. 'Not much of a conversationalist, are you?' Laura and I exchanged wary glances.

'Is that a cut on your hand, Mrs Wimble?' asked Laura. The pair of mittens she was wearing had a reddish stain seeping through. Mrs Wimble looked at her hand curiously. 'Oh yes,' she eventually answered. 'I cut it on some bushes when I went to pick hawthorn berries this afternoon,' she told her, completely unconcerned.

'This afternoon, Mrs Wimble?' I asked.

'Yes, dear. Isn't that right, Derek? You are working very late, girls, and on a Saturday too.' She started to cough again, bringing up a yellowish phlegm into a dirty handkerchief before sinking into an armchair.

'We like to keep an eye on our favourite patients,' chirruped Laura. 'Now, let me take a look at that hand, Mrs Wimble.' Gently she pulled off the mittens. It was a nasty cut. She opened up her bag and started to dress the wound.

'Do you have the correct time please, Mrs Wimble?' I asked.

'Yes, dear. It's almost midnight. I wonder why the sun is still up. Derek, you're completely wrong. It can't be November. Why, it must be almost the Summer Solstice, just look at the evening sky. I won't be dancing around in the altogether anymore,' laughed Mrs Wimble, pulling up her trouser legs to reveal bruising.

'Have you had a fall, Mrs Wimble?' I ventured.

'A fall, dear?' replied Mrs Wimble, a vacant look spreading across her face.

'Your leg is very bruised.'

She looked down at her leg thoughtfully for a while before looking up. 'Miss Hill, how nice to see you. I wonder if you could take a look at my leg. One of the silly cats got trapped upstairs and I took a tumble down the steps when I carried the stupid thing down.'

I felt her head. She was burning up. 'Of course. I'm going to check you over.'

Poor Mrs Wimble. She really believed the voices on Radio 4 were in the room with us and since the last time I'd seen her she'd lost track of time – the dates and seasons had become completely jumbled up in her head. Here we were on Monday morning in November and she thought it a Saturday night in June.

'She's can't go on like this, Sarah,' said Laura as we sadly walked back to the car.

'I know, that cough sounds like a really bad chest infection. I think that fall has made her confused.'

'Yes, I think you're right.'

'I'll drive back to Totley and fetch Dr Drake. I think she'll need to go to Maidstone General.'

Dr Drake immediately admitted Mrs Wimble to hospital. She was furious. But he had very little option than to call in the environmental health team, who went in mob-handed and threw practically everything away into a large rubbish truck. The RSPCA came and took all the cats away too.

A week later, Mrs Wimble was sent home to Peasblossom. It was clean and quiet and completely unrecognisable to her. Laura and I went together to welcome her home. We bathed her, combed out her long grey hair, put her in a clean nightdress and tucked her into crisp white sheets in a new bed social services had put in the sitting room.

When Laura called in the next morning, Mrs Wimble had passed away in the night. She was the first patient I'd lost since arriving in Totley and I'll never forget her: a woman who lived on her own terms till the very end.

*14*

I was glad to have Hermione with me as we passed through the
huge Gothic entrance of the Royal Courts of Justice on the Strand
with its gleaming white spires. I felt a pang for the East End as my
mind traced the path back from central London to the streets of
Hackney. It was wonderful to be in London again but a day at the
Law Courts could hardly be considered a day out. Hermione
squeezed my arm as we went under the elaborately carved
porches with their threatening iron gates into the echoing Great
Hall.

'Chin up, Sarah. It's always daunting being a witness,' sympathised Hermione. 'I remember my first time I had to keep a hand
on my knees to stop them knocking together in the witness box.
It's such a labyrinth, this place, I always worry I'll still be searching for the courtroom by teatime.'

The court usher checked my name off the list and told us to
wait on a long wooden bench.

'Shouldn't be too long, ladies. It is Mr Justice Dalton's last day
on the bench. He's one of the best. He'll be a great loss to Probate,
Divorce and Admiralty, I can tell you,' the usher informed us with
a touch of pride, thumbing his black robe and rocking back on his
heels.

I felt beyond nervous. I'd barely been able to drink a cup of tea
that morning and I couldn't face breakfast. I was worried I'd say
the wrong thing, that somehow it would get twisted – that I'd let

everyone down. Hermione and Mrs King had told me to stick to the facts and not let the barrister twist my words or get me flustered in his cross-examination. Hermione tried to keep me calm with chat about my birthday; we'd celebrated with a small party at the weekend.

'I did enjoy that red-cabbage dish. You must give the recipe. Etty would lap it up,' Hermione complimented.

'I'm glad you enjoyed it. It was quite a jolly party, wasn't it?' It had been a congenial gathering of Mr and Mrs King, Laura, Hermione and myself. Mrs King had suggested I ask Mr Hopkins the headmaster as well.

'It's a shame Mr Shepherd couldn't make it,' Hermione fished.

'But nice that Mr Hopkins was able to join us,' I parried.

Hermione bit her lip, her eyes bright. 'Yes, nice for Jack King not to be the only man for a change. I thought Mrs Farthing's gift of strawberry wine was a welcome addition.'

'Lethal, wasn't it?'

'It certainly loosened us up a bit,' Hermione said with a chuckle.

We waited for what seemed like an age but was no more than a couple of hours until the usher called my name. I jumped to attention.

'They are all back from lunch. After you've given your testimony, you and your friend can sit in the gallery,' he helpfully informed us.

'All rise for the Honourable Mr Justice Redvers Dalton,' announced the court clerk.

A medium-sized old gentleman in a black robe with golden tabs on each shoulder and a white wig shuffled onto the judge's bench. He took a few moments arranging himself.

'Miss Gamble, your next witness if you please.'

'Miss Sarah Hill, m'lud. Mrs Bunyard's health visitor,' replied the barrister donned in a black gown and crisp white shirt and a short white wig.

Mrs Bunyard gave me a nervous half-smile as I went into the witness box. She was wearing a pale-blue skirt suit with a soft peach blouse. Mr Bunyard sat next to her, holding his wife's hand and looking very smart in a brown suit, with his hair oiled and combed back. I glanced at the other side. A barrister with a beaky nose and narrow eyes sat coolly next to an older lady dressed in tweeds. She had an angular jaw made even more prominent by pulling her grey hair into a tight austere bun. This must be Susan's aunty, Mildred Smith. She didn't look like a woman to be trifled with.

The clerk of the court brought me a Bible and made me swear on it to tell the truth. Miss Gamble rose slowly and walked purposefully over to the witness box. She smiled at me. 'Good afternoon, Miss Hill.'

'Good afternoon.'

'You are my client, Mrs Bunyard's, health visitor, are you not?'

'I am.'

'You've seen first-hand Mrs Bunyard with her younger daughter, Sharon?'

'Yes.'

'From your professional observations would you say Mrs Bunyard is a good mother?'

'Yes, I'd say she is a very caring and dedicated mother.'

'Is she a suitable person for the care and control of a young child?'

'Yes.'

'Do you think she is capable of providing a loving home for a child?'

'Yes, I do.'

'Have you ever had cause to doubt Mrs Bunyard's capabilities of caring for a young child?'

'None at all.'

'Has Mrs Bunyard talked about her elder daughter, Michelle Smith, to you?'

'She has, yes.'

'What has she said to you about Michelle Smith?'

'That she wants to be part of her life. That she regrets giving her up and wants to have contact. To give her a mother's love.'

'A mother's love?'

'Yes.'

'As a health visitor how important is a mother's love to a child?'

'I'd say it was the most important part of their emotional development.'

'But surely anyone can feed and water a child?'

'Well, not anyone.'

'But most people can make meals, change nappies, give a child a bottle of milk, buy clothes, house them?'

'Yes.'

'But what of love?'

'Love is everything to a child. Whether or not your mother loves you and you have access to that love shapes your life.'

'Whether or not your mother loves you shapes your life,' repeated Miss Gamble slowly. 'Would you say Mrs Bunyard is a loving mother?'

'Yes, very loving,' I answered.

'Do other professionals put such emphasis on mother's love or, if you'll forgive me, is it merely the sentimental notion of a very young health visitor?' she asked with a wry smile.

'No. I attended a lecture by Dr Mia Kellmer Pringle, an eminent child psychologist and Director of the National

Children's Bureau only this month. She argues that "mother-love" is unmeasurable. That motherly love in infancy and childhood is as important for mental health as are vitamins and proteins for physical health.'

'Given your belief in the importance of a mother's love to a child like Michelle, my client's beloved daughter, would you say it would be in Michelle's best interests to see her mother?'

'I would say it would benefit her immeasurably.'

'Do you think given time and support Michelle Smith could be part of a loving family with Susan and Alan Bunyard and her baby sister, Sharon?'

'I do, absolutely.'

'Thank you, Miss Hill. No further questions, m'lud,' concluded Miss Gamble.

'Your witness, Mr Morton,' the judge addressed Mrs Smith's barrister.

'Thank you, m'lud. Miss Hill, motherly love is the stuff of sentimental fairy tales, is it not?' advanced Mr Morton.

'No, it's proven that attachment forms a child's psychological development,' I answered guardedly.

'But surely children can form attachments to people other than their mothers?' he tried again.

'Yes, they can.'

'Are you close to your mother, Miss Hill? What about your father – is he so unimportant in your life?'

'Mr Gamble, I do not see what bearing personal questions about this nice lady's private life have on this case,' Mr Justice Dalton refereed. But he had caught me off-balance. I felt a pang of disloyalty to my parents and self-doubt was only inches away.

Mr Morton acknowledged the reprimand with a nod of the head and a quick flash of an insincere smile to me, baring the top and bottom rows of his teeth.

'Miss Hill, is it likely that Michelle Smith, having lived with Mrs Smith, who has been after all her legal custodian since infancy, and for the last three years has to all intents and purposes been her mother, formed an attachment to her loving aunt that is equal to what you sentimentally call "motherly love"?'

'I don't know.'

'You don't know?' he mocked me.

'I've never met Mrs Smith,' I tried to explain.

'You've never met Mrs Smith?' repeated Mr Morton with incredulity. 'Have you ever met Michelle Smith?' he pressed.

'No.'

'Then how can you possibly know whether or not it is best for Michelle Smith to be in the custody of her aunt, who to all intents and purposes is her mother?'

'Because she's not her mother,' I snapped.

'How can you know the damage removing a three-year-old child from the only home she's ever known has? Surely that has psychological implications far beyond a mere health visitor? Let's talk about the impact of being abandoned by your mother. Mrs Bunyard, or Susie Smith as she was then, a callous, unmarried girl, was supposed to love her child above all else, but she didn't. She left her. So tell me, Miss Hill, what about abandonment, does that not have an emotional impact on a child's development?'

I couldn't speak. 'Miss Hill, answer the question.' Mr Morton jabbed at me.

'It can, yes,' I responded. 'Which is why it would be beneficial for Michelle to have contact with her mother so she can know she loves her and wants to be with her,' I pleaded, turning to face the judge.

But Mr Morton had me on the ropes and continued pommelling his point home. 'You expect this court to give contact to a callous young woman who got herself pregnant by a convicted criminal at only 16? Who abandoned her child as soon as she gave birth to her? Never visited or bothered with her. Then, on a whim, this same callous young woman now wants to uproot a defenceless child she doesn't even know from the loving and secure home she enjoys with her aunt, Mildred Smith, who is to all intents and purposes Michelle Smith's mother.'

I didn't know what to say. Was he asking me a question?

'Mr Morton, we both have the social worker's report and recommendations,' the judge intervened. 'Miss Hill is here to talk about the suitability of Mrs Bunyard and her husband as custodians of Mrs Bunyard's child. Please keep your questions appropriate to the witness.'

'I was simply trying to establish that Mrs Smith provides an equally loving and suitable home for Michelle Smith and has been doing so for over three years since the mother abandoned her child, m'lud. The child Mrs Bunyard conceived out of wedlock with a criminal. It is not the stuff of fairy tales,' replied Mrs Smith's beaky barrister.

'Do not make your speeches during cross-examination, Mr Morton,' insisted Mr Justice Dalton. 'I would not want you labouring under the false impression that because it is my last day on the bench I will allow this in my courtroom,' chastised the judge.

'No further questions, m'lud,' replied Mr Morton as he slinked back to his seat.

'Miss Hill,' the judge addressed me, 'have you in your capacity as Mrs Bunyard's health visitor discussed with her why she gave up her child?'

'I have, your lordship.'

'I do not allow hearsay in my court, Miss Hill, but what is your understanding of why Mrs Bunyard neglected this most sacred of responsibilities?' he asked earnestly.

'She told me that she was young and scared. That she had recently lost her own mother. Her boyfriend was sent to prison. She told me she felt alone and had no means to provide for her child. She told me her aunt persuaded her it would be in the child's best interests. She told me her aunt had promised that she would be allowed to be part of her baby's life. I do not believe it was ever Mrs Bunyard's intention to abandon her child. What I do know is that there was no formal adoption. Mrs Bunyard never legally gave up her child. Mrs Smith had possession of Michelle Smith but she did not have Mrs Bunyard's full consent to permanent custody. We can't know what passed between aunt and niece for sure but we do know it was an informal adoption.'

'Thank you, Miss Hill. That is all. You may leave the witness box.'

As I sat with Hermione, I felt momentary relief to leave the witness box but quickly a feeling of reproach overcame me. I had tried to tell the truth, the whole truth and nothing but the truth, but I could have done better. I could have answered better. It didn't matter a jot if I looked inexperienced; in truth I *was* inexperienced. What mattered was getting the best outcome for little Michelle – what if I had in some way jeopardised that and let her down?

Mrs Bunyard and Mrs Smith were both cross-examined before I was allowed into the courtroom. I will never know how Susan fared under Mr Morton's questioning but he had me rattled. Before asking counsel to make their closing arguments the kindly-faced judge asked Michelle Smith's aunt and mother if there was anything they would like to add to their statements and to say to each other.

Mrs Smith turned her frosty gaze onto her niece. 'It's the ingratitude, Susan. We could have sent you to a mother and baby home. We could have given away your child to strangers. I've loved Michelle like she's my own. God never saw fit to give me a child – Michelle is the only chance I'll ever have to be a mother. You're a cruel, cruel heartless girl to want to take her away from me. You've already got a baby and you can go on having them. If Michelle sees you, then who am I? I won't be her mother anymore.'

A pang of sympathy rushed through me for Mrs Smith and I thought of the children I'd seen who really needed loving adoptive parents, whose life chances were greatly improved by being removed, but Michelle Smith was not one of them. She had a loving mother who wanted her and that was priceless.

The judge asked Susan Bunyard if she had anything else to say. She took a moment to steady herself. I could see the quick rise and fall of her chest as she attempted to get her breathing under control as she spoke one last time in court.

'I'm sorry you feel that, Aunty. I'm grateful you cared for Michelle and loved her but I'm married now and Michelle needs to be part of our family,' she replied. 'My little Michelle is always in my thoughts. I've prayed every day since she was born; prayed for her to be happy and content and loved. Even when I thought for a long time she would never know my love I tried to console myself that she would be loved by you, Aunty. But now I'm a little bit older and I know no one can give her the love that I can. Please give me the chance to let her know I love her. She might never forgive me for giving her up – it was never my plan to leave her, it just happened. Don't you remember, Aunty, you came with me to the hospital when I had her? You told me Michelle would know I was her mummy but that changed overnight. Before I knew what was what, you'd taken the baby home with you. I didn't want to give my baby away – you made that decision for me. I should have stood up to you but I didn't know how. For a year I would wake up in the night and think my baby was crying for me. I wanted to run to her. I wanted to run barefoot in my nightdress to your house and take her back every single night. I cried myself to sleep every night until I went to Kent and met Ally. And for the longest time it felt like there was no way back.

'When I got married and had Sharon I couldn't push it down anymore. Sharon wasn't a replacement for Michelle. You can't replace one child for another. I want both my children. I don't want to lie to either of my daughters. I'm proud to have brought both of them into this world. I don't want Michelle to be a lie, to be a source of shame – she's a joy to me. I want us to be a family. Michelle is innocent in this – she's only a baby really, please, she deserves to be loved by her mum. I was a silly girl. I did get pregnant by a no-good thief, but I didn't know then – I thought I was in love, I couldn't say no to him. But I've pulled myself together. We can give Michelle a loving home.

'Ally's got a loan to fix up our cottage. We're going to make it lovely. I'm getting a room ready for Michelle because she'll always be welcome. Charlie Carter is not going to be her father. He's not registered on her birth certificate. He's got no rights to her. I know he'll try and get her. Aunty, we need to work together to keep Michelle safe. Let me see her, oh, let me see her. Let me protect her. You won't be here for ever – what will happen to Michelle then?' she pleaded, one hand pressed to her chest, the other gripping the wooden table to steady herself as a torrent of regret, shame, hope and fear overwhelmed her.

'Counsel, if you'd like to prepare your closing remarks,' invited the judge.

'Thank you, m'lud,' began Miss Gamble. 'This case is for you to decide whether a three-year-old child, Michelle Smith, should have the right to see her mother.' She touched Mrs Bunyard's shoulder. 'I put it to you that Susan Bunyard is a loving mother. A caring and capable person who dearly wants to be part of her daughter's life. That has been supported both in her own testimony and the evidence from her health visitor and the Children's Department. The report confirms that Susan Bunyard should be granted not only access but ultimately transferred care and control of her beloved daughter.

'Michelle Smith was informally adopted by her great-aunt, Mrs Smith. Susan Bunyard did not want to give up her baby; she has been separated from her and now wishes to ensure that her child knows she is loved. Throughout history and literature children have been stolen, adopted and brought up by adults who are not their biological parents. A statute of Moses in this great building reminds us of this. When the Pharaoh ordered all Hebrew baby sons to be thrown into the Nile, Moses' mother in order to try and save her baby hid him in the bulrushes in a basket. The Pharaoh's daughter found him, and he became her son and she called him Moses. But divine provenance brought the baby back to his own mother and sister. Our parents give us the key to our identity. A mother's love is priceless.

'Michelle Smith is not Jane Eyre. There is no need for her to be separated from her mother. M'lud, you can today bestow this gift and reunite mother and child,' encouraged Miss Gamble.

She then opened a box on her table and brought out a pair of small pink leather shoes. Just the right size for a three-year-old girl. 'I ask you, m'lud, to put yourself in Michelle Smith's shoes. Wouldn't you want to be with your mummy?' concluded Miss Gamble.

Hermione and I both looked at each other, blinking back tears of faith and approbation. I couldn't really listen to most of Mr Morton's speech. I couldn't stop thinking about those pink shoes, that small baby taken away from her mummy, and I ached with it all. I only heard Mr Morton's final remarks.

'My learned friend mentioned Jane Eyre and Moses,' he scoffed. 'Moses was raised as a prince rather than a slave. And as for Jane Eyre, Mrs Smith is not a neglectful guardian but a most loving and lawful custodian of this child. Michelle Smith knows no other mother,' he concluded.

Mrs Smith nodded approvingly but she looked pale and hot. I noticed her trying to catch her breath several times during the afternoon. It was a November day and yet the old lady was constantly wiping her brow with a lace-trimmed handkerchief. I pitied her. What would happen to Michelle if something happened to her guardian and she'd never known her mother? Yes, it would mean Mrs Bunyard would get custody but they would be strangers – we didn't want that.

The judge was silent and we all waited. Would he make a decision there and then, or call a break to consider? He arranged his face into a serious but kindly manner and began.

'On the bench there are judges who doubt the practical and moral characters of mothers who have children outside of wedlock. I may have been born in the eleventh hour of Queen Victoria's reign but to me that is one moral judgement that should be left in the past. As counsel points out, throughout history children have been raised by people who are not their natural parents with mixed results. I judge it would not be in the best interests of Michelle Smith to suddenly remove her from a home she has been in for more than three years, morally, psychologically or in accordance with The Children Act 1975. Under section 35 the child's mother, Mrs Susan Bunyard, is petitioning for access with a view to custody after having access denied by her aunt, Mrs Smith, the child's legal custodian. The evidence shows that Mrs Bunyard is not a neglectful mother. She has had three years to mature and understand that actions have consequence. But what are the consequences of the time mother and child have spent apart? Is it fair on Michelle Smith to reunite her with a woman she does not know and tell her this is in fact her mother? What would Michelle gain from this?

'Mrs Bunyard is not an abusive or neglectful woman, she poses no threat to the child, but revocation of legal custodianship is not something one rushes into lightly. The reports from the Children's Department in Essex where the child is resident show that she is well cared for. There is also the impeding issue of the father's rights, which will need to be dealt with as and when a legal application is made. I am not granting transfer of guardianship today from Mrs Smith to Mrs Bunyard. But with immediate effect Mrs Smith must give Mrs Bunyard access to her child for specified times. For the next six months Mrs Bunyard can visit her daughter on alternate Saturdays in Essex. These visits do not need to be supervised and Mrs Bunyard is free to take the child out if that is her preference.

'After six months the court will reconvene to hear the professional reports on the effect the relationship has had on the child – unless Mrs Bunyard and Mrs Smith can come to an arrangement themselves before that time. Mrs Smith, I do sympathise with your situation but eventually I believe the courts will transfer custody to your niece. Coming to an amicable arrangement before the six months is up would be better for you all and especially Michelle,' ruled the judge.

'All rise, Mr Justice Dalton,' announced the court clerk. We were all swiftly on our feet as the benevolent judge exited his courtroom one last time.

'Are you happy now, Susie?' shouted Mrs Smith.

I watched Susan nervously cross the court to face up to her red-cheeked aunt.

'You don't look very well, Aunty.'

'Not well. You're killing me, you wicked girl,' snapped Mrs Smith. Her body was trembling with rage.

'I know it's hard, but I'd like to take you to tea now and talk about what we tell Michelle and how best we can make this work.'

'I hope you choke on your tea,' wished her aunt before she started to cry into her handkerchief with big heaving sobs, her rigid body suddenly rippled with emotion. Susan reached out her arms, held her aunt and let her cry. Mildred Smith's hot salty tears left watermarks on her niece's blouse and jacket.

'Come on,' Hermione nudged me. 'I'll treat you to tea at The Savoy – it's only a hop, skip and a jump.'

I followed her obediently back through the passages and tunnels that led out into the twilight of the Strand. Suddenly, the cold air hit my face and I felt momentarily giddy and then exhilarated to be outside, in London, free from the solemnity of the courthouse and the responsibility of the witness box. Susan had won. She was going to get back the baby she thought she'd lost, I knew she would.

I linked arms with Hermione. We paraded down the street, carried on a whirlwind of triumph through the roar of the traffic, the twinkling of street lights and the glorious sight of London red buses bustling up and down the Strand.

The doorman held open the door for us. 'Never mind tea, let's live dangerously and have a cocktail at the American Bar,' said Hermione. And before I knew it she had the bartender eating out of the palm of her hand. My glamorous pal was laughing gaily then all of a sudden her face dropped as she gazed over my shoulder. I followed her gaze and there in a corner of the bar drinking champagne like butter wouldn't melt was Nick Shepherd with a smartly dressed girl. It took me a moment and then I realised it was Felicity Bourne, the Bishop's daughter.

'Do you want to go?' asked Hermione.

'Why should we?' I replied, flicking my long dark hair haughtily over my shoulder. 'We aren't going out you know.'

'I know, but I thought …'

'Well, so did I. But there you go.'

I looked once more at the pair of them, thick as thieves. Nick glanced up and caught my eye. Mr Smooth started shifting about uncomfortably in his tight suit, a pink rash spreading up from underneath his dog collar to his earlobes. He looked at me desperately with those huge dark eyes. I almost felt sorry for catching him out. Felicity clocked me and Hermione at the bar. With a satisfied air she took Nick firmly by the hand and pulled him with her as she bounced up to the bar.

'Isn't it wonderful? We're engaged!' she burst out, flashing a sapphire engagement ring on her finger.

'When was this?' asked Hermione.

'Just now. Do you like my ring? It was my grandmother's. I picked it up from our safety deposit box this afternoon – isn't it a coincidence?' she said with a titter.

'Mr Shepherd, you asked Miss Bourne to marry you in The Savoy, how romantic,' Hermione purred.

Nick said nothing.

'We decided it was about time, didn't we, Nicholas?' Felicity informed us.

Nick nodded. He gulped, a lump protruding in his throat.

'Totley Parsonage is in desperate need of a woman's touch,' Hermione suggested.

'Oh no! I don't think we'll stay in sleepy Totley. Daddy's got big plans for Nicholas.'

'Marvellous. Have you set a date yet?' teased Hermione.

'Canterbury Cathedral on 7 June,' answered Felicity.

'Goodness, you are organised,' complimented Hermione.

'You have to be. If I left it to Nicholas I doubt we'd ever make it up the aisle,' she said, laughing loudly.

'I don't know about you, Hermione, but I fancy a night out in Chinatown,' I said. I'd had enough of Felicity already.

'Rather,' Hermione agreed, sipping the last of her cocktail.

'Oh yes, and we must get back. My brother Peter is coming to celebrate with us, and Daddy's at Lambeth Palace at some ecclesiastical borefest. I'm going to powder my nose. Good evening, Miss Drummond, and, er, I don't know your name?'

Nick finally found his voice. 'It's Miss Hill, Felicity.'

Felicity gave me a smug smile and then sauntered off to the ladies' loos without saying goodbye.

'Sarah, I …' started Nick.

'There's no need to explain. Congratulations.'

Hermione and I linked arms once more and embarked on the bright lights of the city.

'I'm sorry, Sarah,' she whispered.

'Don't be. We never really got started and I'm pretty sure Felicity Bourne had booked Canterbury Cathedral before I even arrived in Totley,' I said.

# 15

All was not well at Hollow Prospect. I'd been visiting Valerie Milstead every two weeks for three months and I felt more like a milk-delivery service than a health visitor. She didn't trust me – I spent most of the visits biting my lip to stop asking too many questions, or listening, really listening, my ears ready to prick up at the slightest hint that she needed help, but she didn't say a word. Some weeks Valerie was chatty; like any teenage girl she was interested in fashion, music and film stars. Other days she was cross and took the milk with barely a word. I was in and out again in under five minutes.

Each market day Valerie seemed a little older and rougher round the edges. The work of caring for her two uncles and the baby in their Victorian household was too much for any girl. That day she looked pale and withdrawn and with good reason.

'Thanks for waiting in the lane till they'd gone. They took their time this morning. Wanted serving up the works before they went in that old banger to market,' explained Valerie as I held baby Mikey while she washed up with water from the copper hopper in the laundry. It was a cold wet December day and Miss Milstead's prospects didn't seem to be on the up.

We spent 10 minutes saying barely a word before she confided, 'They're cross with me.'

'Why?' I asked levelly. It didn't pay to probe too much with Valerie.

'Because I insisted they take us to hospital on Saturday night. I thought Mikey was gonna stop breathing, his chest was so bad. That room is like an icicle – your breath mists in front of you.'

'It must have been frightening for you,' I sympathised.

'It was awful. Mikey woke me in the night. He made this funny noise and then he couldn't get his breath. I was so scared, I started screaming. My uncles came banging on the door. I thought they were going to break it down.'

'Had you locked it?'

'I put a chair against the handle,' she continued quickly before I could ask another question. 'They didn't want to take him to hospital but I wouldn't take no for an answer and said I'd run to a payphone and call an ambulance. They didn't want that so they took me to Maidstone General.'

Valerie Milstead turned to face the wall again as she washed.

'I don't like hospitals much either. It was nicer on the maternity ward. Have you been in hospitals a lot?' she asked, changing the subject.

'Yes, Miss Milstead. I'm a nurse. I trained and worked in a hospital.'

'Would you call me Valerie? I never hear my name any more.'

'If you like.' Then I tried, 'What do your uncles call you?'

'Girl.' There was a long pause. 'The doctor was so snooty,' she continued. 'It was horrible. He said I didn't look after Mikey properly, said he was "underfed". I told him, "Mikey has plenty of National Dried" and he looked down his nose at me and said, "I'd expect nothing less." My uncles wouldn't even come in – they stayed in the car park. I was all on my own.'

Valerie went quiet and still for a moment or two before pressing on with the washing-up with renewed vigour.

'Did you bring me some more National Dried?' she asked.

'Yes, I'll get it in a sec. What else did the doctor say?'

'He said Mikey needed feeding up. Should I be giving him real food already?'

'Do you think he's ready?'

'He seems happy enough. I'm sure he'll pipe up when he's ready. When he does come off the bottle you won't be coming every week with the milk, will you?' she concluded.

'I can still come if you'd like me to, Valerie.'

'Why? Do you think I don't know what I'm doing too?'

'No, I think you're doing well. You're working so hard all the time.'

'I never get a minute.'

'I know, it's very hard.'

'More hard than you know.'

She stopped washing up. I stood next to her and put my hand on her shoulder.

'I'm always here if you need anything or you want to talk,' I said gently.

'They'll be back soon. Can I have that milk before you go, please, Nurse? I've saved up my tokens.'

The visit was over. What was going on? Please tell me, Valerie, please, I thought, as I drove off with nothing to report, nothing to do. Only awful suspicions that for her sake I hoped weren't true. Valerie was never going to divulge her full story, and I worried that if I pushed too hard she'd tell me to clear off and never come back. This was the worst part of my job and I felt useless.

I drove on to my next visit. Fat lot of use you'll be when you get there, I reproached myself.

The afternoon sun had battled through the cloud and was getting low over the bare orchards of Mill Farm, turning the skyline a russet hue. My little green Mini trundled over Station Bridge to the other side of the tracks – the wrong side of the tracks, Flo would say. I had a primary visit to do on a 10-day-old baby at the gypsy camp that was lodged at Mill Farm for the winter. Flo had remarked they lowered the tone of the village but Clem told me they'd been coming to Totley every winter since his grandfather's day and Sid Holleman the farmer swore they brought good luck and blessed the orchards. I followed the track until it became a mud path, a mire of large wheeled tracks and horses' hooves. There was nothing for it but to pull on my wellies and make my way on foot.

I looked up at the sky. It would probably be dark by the time I came back and I hadn't brought a torch. Another piece of equipment they don't issue on the NHS for community nurses, I thought. I frowned, how far would it be to the campsite? Would I get lost in the woods overnight? A little shiver ran through me.

'Is that you, Nurse?' I heard a cheerful voice call. It was Sid Holleman. He jumped down from his red tractor and strode across to meet me.

'Yes, afternoon, Mr Holleman. I'm visiting the gypsy camp but I've not been before and I'm wondering if I'll get there and back before dark.'

'I've got a spare torch in the tractor – two ticks,' he reassured me, jogging back to retrieve it. 'It's got plenty of battery. I'll walk you over to the camp now. Don't want you getting lost now, do we?'

'That would be fab, yes, please,' I eagerly replied, and with considerable relief I followed him through the wood at the edge of the orchard. 'Clem says the gypsies come here every winter.'

'Yes, they've been coming since my grandfather's day. There's a dozen caravans but only one of them's a proper Romany wagon; rest of 'em are all modern, like you get on the holiday parks in Herne Bay or Whitstable. When I was a boy they were all proper ones pulled by horses. We had to give 'em three fields for the grazing – they've got a way with horses, the gypsies. But the caravans are all mechanised now, like farming,' he said with a sigh. 'You can't blame 'em. I wouldn't want to swop my tractor for a dray horse. I'll leave you at the gate, Nurse. The camp's in that little copse. Keep the torch,' he finished, before quickly making his way back to his trailer to get as much done as possible before we lost the light.

As soon as I opened the gate several dogs started barking at me. I edged my way round them attempting a steely gaze and indifferent air. A large iron pot and a kettle were hanging on a long stick over a fire. Round it sat several old women on low wooden stools in headscarves and layers of woollens, peeling potatoes and singing in a low tune as a young lad played on a penny whistle. The caravans were dotted around the site but at the centre was an old-fashioned wagon with wooden steps leading to a closed blue door with marvellous gold etchings. Two horses tied up on ropes grazed on the short winter grass next to the caravan while a well-built middle-aged man brushed a golden palomino filly with white patches and a long creamy coloured fringe until she shone. Her companion, a grey mare, tried to nuzzle the palomino out of the way to get the best of the grass. The man looked up at me. Under each dark hooded eye was a deep hollow. Beneath his long grey moustache were pale pink lips that opened up into a broad smile, crinkling up his tanned freckled face. Thick grey wavy locks stuck out in all directions from below a battered red cap, and a scarlet handkerchief was tied in a knot at his neck. He wore no shirt, just a black jacket over a grey vest and ragged-legged trousers tucked into a good pair of sooty boots. It was a pleasant face.

'Can I help you, missus?' he enquired in a low calm tone as he continue to brush his horse.

'Yes, I'm the health visitor. I'm here to see Mrs Drury,' I replied, making my way gingerly through the strewn pots, cups, stools and wooden cabinets towards the pretty little wagon.

'That's our Lisa-Rose. She's next door. Her mammy's taking care of her,' he informed me, nodding in the direction of a sparkling new caravan to the right of the wagon. 'She's not feeling herself,' he added in a confidential tone.

I thanked him and knocked. An older woman opened the door and leant out. She had long raven hair held back by a crimson-and-white spotted handkerchief.

'Who's this, Moses?' she called over my head to her husband.

'It's the nurse, come to see Lisa-Rose,' he reassured her.

'You'd better come in, missus,' she suggested kindly but her face looked concerned. 'I'm Queenie Dangerfield, I'm the granny. We had a bit of bother with the baby but she's right as rain now. Lisa-Rose is having a lie-down. Go through and take a look at her would you, missus.'

It wasn't a big home but it was very comfortable. A shining little palace with beautiful pieces of pottery and porcelain on fine lace cloths. Lisa-Rose was dozing on the bed, her baby nestled next to her. I asked her if the doctor had been to see her that day. She exchanged a quick look with her mother.

'He came two days ago,' she replied carefully.

'How are you feeling, Mrs Drury?' I asked. She looked worryingly pale.

'I'm so tired, missus. I feel wiped out. I feel like a ghost. I've pains in my leg.'

'Can I take a look at your leg, please?'

'Here, Ma, take the baby,' said Lisa-Rose, passing little Fiance to her granny. Agonisingly slowly she pulled back the cover and lifted her leg out with strain before lying back on the pillows, her long black hair spread out. She was a beautiful girl with big brown eyes that widened as my hands touched her leg and she gasped, her finger clutching the gold necklaces she wore in layers round her throat. The leg was hot, swollen and tender; it was twice the size of the other leg and there was a rash in the crook of her knee. She had a temperature. This was not good. I composed my face and said as calmly as I could: 'I'm concerned about your leg, Mrs Drury. If it's all right with you I'm going to walk back to the road and find a payphone and call the doctor. We need to check you haven't got deep vein thrombosis.'

'Is that dangerous?' asked Queenie Dangerfield, looking alarmed.

'If untreated there's a risk of a pulmonary embolism. That's a blockage, usually a blood clot that can stop the blood getting to the heart and lungs. Have you had any difficulty breathing or chest pain, Mrs Drury?'

'No, I haven't.'

'That's good. Shall I go and call the doctor?'

'Please, missus,' replied Lisa-Rose, closing her eyes once more.

I hurried back to my car and drove to the red phone box and dialled. The sun had almost set – I was glad of Sid Holleman's torch.

'Totley Doctors' Surgery,' answered the shrill voice of Miss Barrow the receptionist.

'I need a doctor to come out immediately to the gypsy camp at Mill Farm and see a new mother,' I told her.

'Doctor's busy now and not to be disturbed. Can't she wait?' she enquired churlishly.

'No, she can't wait,' I snapped.

'I can't get hold of Dr Botten on a golf course so she'll have to.'

'Oh, forget it,' I snarled, hanging up the receiver and picking it up again to dial 999.

It was getting dark and there were no signposts. I'd told the operator I'd park my Mini at the end of the lane with my lights on. I waited and waited, sitting there on my tod, my worries increasing as night fell. Where were they? Didn't they know every second counted?

I thought of Lisa-Rose's beautiful face and her hair spread out on the pillow and remembered the mother we'd lost at Hackney during my obstetrics training; the girl I'd never forget. She'd started hyperventilating with a pulmonary embolism – no one had picked up the blood clot. The memory of her still brought tears to my eyes; even now I could see her in her short multi-coloured nightie, her long beautiful black hair spread on the pillow just like Lisa-Rose. Having to pack up her things and give her wedding band in a brown envelope to her grief-stricken husband and watch him kiss her cold body goodbye as I held their tiny motherless new baby in my arms was one of the worst moments of my life. That was not going to happen again – not tonight, not to Lisa-Rose. I prayed over and over again for the ambulance to hurry up but it took over an hour.

The ambulance followed my Mini until I could go no further. I pulled up and hopped in next to the driver and guided them as best I could towards the camp. The fog lights eventually fell on the little campsite and we parked at the gate. A clutch of children were gathered round the campfire eating bowls of stew from a big black cauldron. They looked up like startled deer in the head-lights before some ran, others froze and one lad who'd been play-ing the penny whistle earlier strode over, full of confidence, though he was only about eight.

'We haven't done nothing,' the boy shouted. 'I'm starting school next week so you can clear off.' In the dark he'd mistaken the ambulance for a police van.

Moses Dangerfield intervened. 'Out of the way, Billy-Boy,' he said, nudging the lad aside.

I ran over to breathlessly explain the intrusion. 'I'm sorry, Mr Dangerfield. I've had to call an ambulance to take Lisa-Rose to hospital.'

He scowled and for a moment I felt a little afraid. He said nothing but turned on his heels to guide the ambulance men to the Drurys' caravan.

'They don't like hospitals,' whispered the ambulance driver to me.

'No, but we have a soft spot for nurses,' added Moses Dangerfield. Even in the dusk I could see the ambulance man's face had turned pink. 'You two can wait outside. Go in, missus,' he said firmly.

Quickly, I explained to Lisa-Rose that I'd not been able to get hold of Dr Botten and I know it seemed a bit dramatic but we did need to get her to hospital to be examined.

'It's all right, missus,' she told me softly. 'I want to go to hospital, I know something's not right. Here, Mammy, help make me decent. You can tell them ambulance fellas to wait outside.'

I helped Queenie Dangerfield dress her daughter and wrap up the baby for the journey.

'In truth I'm glad it's not that Dr Botten,' remarked Lisa-Rose.

'Oh yes?' I raised an enquiring eyebrow.

'When he came two days ago he fell down the steps of the caravan. I knew as soon as I looked at him that he was drunk,' she told me.

I glanced at Queenie Dangerfield. She confirmed her daughter's account and added, 'He gave us a bottle of something nasty for the baby. We didn't trust him so we threw it away. I've kept the bottle, though.' Queenie retrieved the medicine from a cabinet. 'Here, look for yourself, missus. He gave us this because the baby had a runny poo. I said to Lisa-Rose they all do that, you no sooner put it into 'em than it shoots out the other end.'

I looked at the bottle: '*Mist. Kaolin and Morph*'. My goodness, that was morphine.

'You did right to throw it away.'

Mrs Dangerfield touched my hand. 'But I can tell you, there's going to be someone up high you'll argue with and you're going to come off the worse for it,' she foretold.

I think you can count on that, Mrs Dangerfield, I pondered as I watched Lisa-Rose, Queenie and baby Fiance climb into the back of the ambulance before it drove off into the night.


'What's all this rubbish?' sniffed Mrs Jefferies, picking up an evergreen woollen ball from my desk.

'It's for my Mothers' Interest Group this morning,' I explained, hastily snatching back the wool and packing it with card, crepe paper, scissors, ribbons and cellophane into a cardboard box.

'Oh, *that*,' Mrs Jefferies sniffed loudly and pulled a face like there was a bad smell in the room. 'I really don't see how that has anything to do with community health. Perhaps you'd have been more suited to being a primary school teacher. I said as much to Miss Presnell last week ...'

Had she indeed! Surprise, surprise. 'I didn't think you came to the clinic on Mondays?' I rapidly attempted to change the subject.

'I don't usually. But Miss Presnell asked to see me. She likes to chew over issues with me from time to time. I *am* the most long-serving member of the health-visiting team.'

Flo bustled in, her arms full of groceries. 'Here's the desiccated coconut, icing sugar and tins of condensed milk you wanted,' she said cheerily. 'Do you want a hand carrying it all over to the church hall?'

'Thanks, Flo. No, I can manage.' I popped them into the box too.

'Are you opening a cake shop?' Mrs Jefferies asked, poking through the box. She located packets of marshmallows that were Christmas treats for the children and without asking opened a pack and started to pop the pink and white confection into her mean mouth one by one.

My phone rang. Mrs Jefferies reached over to answer it but I got in quick and picked up the receiver myself.

'Totley Health Visitors, Sarah Hill speaking,' I answered.

'Dr Botten wants to see you right away,' instructed Miss Barrow with no introduction.

'I've got my mothers' interest group in half an hour,' I replied.

'Well, you'd better get a move on then,' she informed me and true to form she hung up abruptly before I could say anything else.

Dr Botten was sitting at his large desk with his palms stretched out, pressing down on either side of his blotter, a single letter in front of him. He didn't ask me to take a seat and I stood before him like a third former sent to the head teacher's office. He savoured the moment and a pregnant pause fell over us before he began to explain why I'd been summoned.

'I've had a letter from the paediatric consultant about the Milstead baby. He was referred for breathing difficulties.' He put on a pair of spectacles and glanced over the missive though clearly he was already familiar with its contents.

'Yes, I have raised my concerns with you about Michael Milstead's breathing due to the conditions in the house on several occasions, Dr Botten.' I tried to keep the irritation out of my voice.

'Are you a doctor now?' he barked, slamming the letter back down on the desk.

'No.'

'Don't interrupt.' His face was reddening and he took a quick swig from a hip flask to regain his composure. His eyes were over-bright and he stared wildly at the letter. 'Imagine my surprise this morning when I got this letter informing me that you've never even clapped eyes on the Milstead child.'

'What? I'm baffled, I don't understand it. I've been seeing Miss Milstead and her baby fortnightly for months.' What was he on about? Was he still sozzled from the night before?

'Have you indeed?' he snorted. 'Well, that's the problem with you community nurses, we never really know where you are, do we? You say you're out on visits but you could be shopping in Tunbridge Wells for all we know. Or making unsavoury friends with little tell-tales at the gypsy camp.' His eyes darkened. 'The paediatrician was as shocked as I am that you should fail in your duties to help such a vulnerable mother and child.' He got to his feet and came round the desk, reading the letter with relish. 'The paediatrician says and I quote: "Get the idle health visitor to visit mother and baby to advise on feeding, care and general management."' He finished by thrusting the letter in my face with a satisfied smirk.

I looked at the letter. 'That's simply not true. I shall write to him myself and put him in the picture.'

'Do you think consultants read correspondence from mere health visitors?' He paused, savouring his triumph. 'I have of course already informed Miss Presnell.' He returned to his desk and picked up his paperwork without giving me another look.

'That is all, Miss Hill.' He dismissed me.

My mouth fell open, but no words came out. I turned on my heels and marched back up Totley Hill. I will not cry, I will not cry on the street, I repeated to myself. I forced myself to return cheery cries of 'Good morning, Nurse' with smiles and enquiries into people's weekend activities and general health all the time wondering why would Valerie Milstead tell the paediatrician she'd never seen a health visitor – why would she do that to me? The next day was the Tuesday cattle market and I'd see her as I always flaming did and ask her what she was playing at.

'Now, ladies,' I said with my brightest smile. 'Today we are going to be making coconut ice,' I informed the gathering of mums assembled for the Monday morning Mothers' Interest Group. The toddlers were playing with toys at the back of the church hall and I had to speak up to be heard over their joyful cries as they discovered my stash of red crepe paper and tissue. Flo had come with me despite my protests and I was grateful to her now, as I watched her, mother-hen like, cluck over the children as they made pompoms to hang on the Christmas tree. Several little ones were already tangled up in the wool full of the excitement of festive preparations; their laughter was soothing. I felt my heart lift for a moment before a side door edged open and my manager, Miss Presnell, emerged and sat quietly at the back of the hall. She'd never been before and gave no explanation for her presence. Each mum was watching me, waiting for me to begin. My mums had donned aprons and assembled before tables laid out with ingredients, small boxes and cellophane.

'Today we will be making coconut ice,' I repeated. 'It's an inexpensive treat to give to a neighbour or relative, or for you to enjoy in front of the telly on Christmas Day with your feet up,' I suggested. 'Let's start. Take your bowl and put in six ounces of icing sugar. No need to weigh as I've measured it all out for you, and there'll be a recipe card for each of you to take home at the end.' I felt like Delia Smith as I explained and demonstrated the recipe. 'Pour in the whole tin of condensed milk and mix it together with a wooden spoon.'

'I love this stuff,' shouted Jackie Bowyer. 'I could drink it out of the tin.'

'It wouldn't do much for your figure,' teased Carol Mires.

'It's all right. My Trev's always preferred a curvier woman,' hooted Jackie. 'I've seen him eyeing up the midwife when she calls many a time.'

I bet Delia doesn't get this, I thought as I waited for the tittering to tail off. 'Stir in five ounces of desiccated coconut. When it's completely mixed divide into two halves and transfer one half to your second bowl.'

'Whoops!' screamed Carol. 'Nurse, I've dropped mine on the floor,' she cried. A big dollop of sticky mixture had splattered onto the dusty floor next to her beautiful red court shoes.

'Don't worry, Mrs Mires. Divide it again so you can have a go with the remaining mixture and you can have mine at the end.'

Carol grinned as she scooped up the mess. Her twins were lying on a blanket at her feet and one had already stuck a podgy hand in and was licking it off his fingers. I looked away.

'She gets extra for being a butter fingers – that's not fair, Nurse,' teased Jackie.

'Sssh,' scolded Susan Bunyard. 'Carry on, Nurse,' she encouraged. There was another fit of giggles.

'Add a few drops of cochineal to one half.'

'Cock-a-what?' whooped Jackie. 'And you're such a lady, Nurse.'

'What's gotten into you this morning, Jackie?' Susan Bunyard interrupted. 'Have you broken open the Advocaat early?'

'It's pink food colouring,' I explained patiently. 'Take the cochineal and add it to one half of the mixture and stir it in.'

Carol dipped in a finger. 'It tastes lovely, Nurse. I think even I could manage this on my own.'

'I'm glad to hear it, Mrs Mires. Once it's mixed in, take your small Tupperware box and put the white mixture on the base and press in,' I said, demonstrating. The room was now momentarily quiet with concentration. 'Once you've pressed it down, add the pink mixture on top and press the two halves firmly together. Write your names on the stickers and put it on the lid of the box. Give them all to me. I'll put them in the fridge. When you get home, cut it up into little squares and put it back in the fridge. If you want to give them to friends, you can make up small gifts by placing the cubes into the centre of the cellophane circles I've cut out for you and tie up with the ribbon,' I suggested, lifting up a cellophane circle and piece of string. 'Why not use the front of the Christmas cards people gave you last year by cutting them into little squares and using as gift tags?'

They all industriously sealed the lids of their Tupperware as directed and brought them to the front.

'A lovely gift and it just takes a few pence and a little bit of effort,' I finished, collecting up the boxes to put in the big fridge in the kitchen. 'They'll keep in the fridge for two to three weeks,' I added as I backed through the double doors laden with sweets.

When I returned, the mums were eating a tray of coconut ice I'd made up the night before for the demonstration.

'You don't mind, do you, Nurse?' said Mrs Underwood with a mouthful.

'Not at all. Let's have some coffee now. Then after our break the children can help us make decorations for the tree and house.'

'You are clever, Nurse,' complimented Susan. 'It's going to be a lovely Christmas and look really festive without me having to put it all on tick.'

I smiled. My eyes searched out the figure of Miss Presnell at the back of the hall. She was writing into a small notebook with a pencil, her forehead furrowed and her mouth turned down. My manager didn't say a word to me for a whole two hours. At lunchtime, once all the mothers had left and Flo and I were tidying up, she came forward.

'Can I get you anything, Miss Presnell?' asked Flo.

'I would like a dozen of your excellent eggs if you can spare them, Mrs Farthing,' she answered. 'Could I collect them from you at the clinic in about 20 minutes? This won't take long.'

'Of course, I'll get them for you now. If that's all right with you, Miss Hill?'

'Yes, thank you for your help today,' I answered.

Flo hurried off. Miss Presnell inspected my box of left-over ingredients and odds and ends of paper.

'I've been meaning to see how your group was going for some time, Miss Hill.' I gulped. 'It's quite a jolly affair, isn't it? Make, do and mend, cooking family meals on a budget, craft and chat – is that what you're doing here?'

'I think that's a fair assessment, Miss Presnell.'

'Sort of thing we learned from our mothers if we were lucky enough,' she suggested.

'Perhaps.'

'Not strictly health work though, is it?'

'It's preventative,' I chirped up.

'Indeed?' She raised one eyebrow curiously. 'Making sweets is work for dentists, I suppose,' she mused with a wry smile.

'That's because it's Christmas. Usually, we look at things like how to make family food on a budget, or buying bigger clothes for the children, and taking them up and letting them down bit by bit so they last longer. I'm planning on a make-up lesson with one of the girls from the department store in Maidstone.'

'Explain yourself if you would, Miss Hill.'

'Eating better has an impact on your health. But so does feeling better. If our homes are nice, if our clothes are smart, if we know a few tricks to present ourselves to the world without spending too much, doesn't it make us feel better – happier? It's not just the skills but getting together, knowing there are people you can talk to if you need to. Mums can feel really isolated here. Not just when they are in the middle of nowhere but if they're new to the area, or feel trapped – being at home with children all day isn't easy. When it's winter you can't even go to the park,' I answered her hopefully.

'I agree, Miss Hill.'

'You do?'

'Oh yes. Health is more than viruses and diseases. We are complicated beings. A healthy mother and baby is more than immunisations and growth checks. You carry on with your group, Miss Hill. I think you're doing a marvellous job.'

'Thank you, Miss Presnell.'

'Now about this other matter. Dr Botten telephoned me at home quite inappropriately at seven o'clock this morning. I thought there'd been some sort of disaster. I think the best course of action would be for me to return to the clinic and see your records of visits to Miss Milstead.'

'Certainly, Miss Presnell.'

We walked together silently along the main road back to the clinic. Grateful the office was empty, I unlocked my filing cabinet and handed Miss Presnell Michael Milstead's records. She took a seat at my desk and read through them diligently without a word. I stood and waited until she had finished and handed the records back to me.

'You've been visiting a little too often in my opinion, but I'll leave that to you. There's no complaint to answer. I didn't think there would be. Do you think you can continue to work with Dr Botten? It's not much more than snide remarks but I'll take it up for you if you wish, Miss Hill. I don't like doctors making false allegations about my girls.'

I was staggered. Could I work with *him*? I thought for a moment. 'Please don't take it up, Miss Presnell. Valerie Milstead has enough to cope with and I don't see how we could resolve it without distressing her. I intend to get to the bottom of it but in my own way.'

'Well, if that's your decision, I'll be off. As I said, you're doing a marvellous job – carry on.'

'Miss Presnell, there is something else.'

'Yes, Miss Hill?'

'I visited a new mother last week. Her baby had runny stools and Dr Botten prescribed kaolin and morph.'

'For a newborn?'

I nodded. 'Luckily the mother had the sense not to give it to the baby and threw it away.'

'Leave it with me, Miss Hill. I'll report it to the chief medical officer.'

'Thank you.'

'For all the good it'll do. He frequents the nineteenth hole too.'

I parked my Mini in a side road near Hollow Prospect and waited for Valerie's uncles to trundle off to market.

She was sulky with me. 'I've had a terrible night. We've been coughing our lungs up till dawn,' she told me as she cradled Mikey in her arms.

I took a deep breath and said as calmly as I could, 'Dr Botten had a letter from the paediatrician at the hospital you saw last week, Valerie.'

She put the baby in a wicker basket and looked out of the window, turning her head away from me, twisting her apron in her little chapped hands. 'Oh, yes,' she answered in a small voice.

'He seems to think I don't visit you.'

'Oh, it was horrible, Nurse,' she turned back to me, her hands pressing on her chest. 'That stuck-up doctor said I don't look after Mikey properly and hadn't the health visitor told me what to do? I didn't want them to take the baby away from me because they thought I couldn't cope,' she said, sobbing pitifully into her apron. 'So, I said I'd never seen a health visitor. I knew you wouldn't mind,' she added, lifting up her pink-cheeked, tear-stained face. 'You don't mind, do you?' she implored, giving me a hopeful smile like a child who's been caught out stealing from the biscuit tin. I couldn't add to her distress.

'No, I don't mind,' I fibbed. 'I won't put the paediatrician in the picture.'

'I knew you'd look out for me.'

'What do you want to do?'

'What do *I* want to do?' She cocked her head to one side and gave me a curious look. We stared at each other for a moment. We three were quite alone and yet she whispered in my ear, 'Can you get me out, Nurse?'

'You want to leave your uncles?' I asked. Valerie replied with the tiniest of nods. 'I could ask Dr Drake if he'd do a joint referral to the Children's Department. Would you like a flat for just you and Mikey in Maidstone?'

'Would I never see my uncles again?'

'Not if you don't want to.'

'Would they have rights to see Mikey?'

'Only fathers have access rights on the whole,' I said.

She looked away. 'There's no father on Mikey's birth certificate.'

'Then no one has any right to him but you,' I told her.

She sighed. 'I don't want him to grow up here. I want him to have a nice normal life.' She reached into the basket and cuddled him tightly.

'You won't get something straight away,' I cautioned her. 'Even in an urgent case it can take a couple of months to find accommodation.'

'Is my case urgent? Do you think we are in danger?' She drew back from me.

'Danger to your health with the damp conditions,' I explained slowly.

She caught my meaning. 'Nothing else? Nothing that would make me look bad, or would make social workers come round?'

'Is there anything else?'

'No, Nurse. Nothing else,' she told me firmly.

'Are you sure, Valerie?'

'I said so, didn't I?' she snapped. 'But I don't have any money. And if I got a job I don't have anyone I can leave Mikey with. That's why I had to come here.'

'We can get you some money. I'm sure you'll get a weekly allowance but unfortunately it will take time.'

'I can wait, if you get me out I can wait. I'll go on scrubbing for them, and cooking and washing and I won't breathe a word. I'll bring Mikey to sleep downstairs by the fire at night to keep us warm and stick a chair under the doorknob if you'll get me out.'

'Get your things. We'll head straight to Totley and get the doctor to refer you for housing. If we hurry, we can get there and back before your uncles get home from market.' And we ran to the car, Valerie holding tightly onto Mikey. Her face had a new glow to it – it was hope.

★  ★  ★

Valerie and I waited in the car until we saw Miss Barrow and Dr Botten leave together for lunch.

'Quick, let's catch Dr Drake before they come back,' I urged.

We snuck into Totley Doctors' Surgery. I tapped on Dr Drake's door and popped my head round. Where was he? He wasn't at his desk. Oh no – we couldn't wait another week, we couldn't waste another minute, we needed to get things moving now.

'Down here, Miss Hill,' echoed his jovial voice. I followed it and found him on the floor with his legs up the wall in a headstand.

'Can you see a baby for me please, doctor?' I requested.

'When, Miss Hill?' he asked.

I closed the door and tipped my head in an attempt to address him the same way up. 'Now if you would, they're in the waiting room.'

Dr Drake sighed and brought his legs down over his head, then rose to his feet full of energy and good humour. He brushed down the sleeves of his shirt before putting his grey suit jacket back on. 'What do you need, Miss Hill?'

'Chest examination for mother and baby and a referral to the Children's Department and housing.'

He polished his spectacles, steaming the glass with the mist of his breath and rubbing them clean with a yellow handkerchief. 'Is there a reason you aren't making the referral yourself?'

'I thought if we did a joint one and flagged it as urgent it would carry more weight, doctor.'

'Who is it?'

'Valerie Milstead's baby, Michael.'

'I don't believe I know her ... Milstead, Milstead,' he tried to recall. 'Aha! Donald and Raymond at that old place, Hollow Prospect, is it?'

'That's right.'

He tapped his head. 'Meditation and yoga keep both body and mind active,' he said with a grin, pushing his glasses up his nose. 'They're a bit of a funny pair, those Milsteads. I didn't think either of them ever married.'

'Valerie is their niece,' I explained.

'I see. Young girl, is she?'

'She is.'

'No chap on the scene?'

'No, doctor.'

'And you think she would be better off somewhere else, do you? Just her and the baby with a regular social security cheque?'

'I am certain of it, doctor.'

'Bring them in. Let's have a look at the little chap and see what we can do.'

I opened the door and called them in. Valerie said barely a word. Dr Drake examined Michael and then his mother.

'It's a damp old place, I expect, Hollow Prospect?' he asked Valerie.

'It is, doctor,' replied Valerie. 'And cold, it's very cold. We've always got a chill.'

'And what about your bedroom?' he enquired.

Valerie looked at me imploringly.

'There's no heating or hot water in the house,' I answered for her. 'Miss Milstead doesn't even have a fire in her bedroom.'

'Dear, dear, dear,' tutted Dr Drake. 'And you'd like a nice new little flat for you and your baby?'

Valerie licked her dry lips and whispered. 'Yes, please.'

'I think it would be for the best, Miss Hill. I can write my two referrals before I go for lunch. You have my full support in this matter.'

'Thank you, doctor,' I smiled. 'Come on, Miss Milstead, I'll run you back to the farm.'

We walked rapidly back to my car. 'How long have we got?' I asked Valerie.

'About a couple of hours,' she answered. 'But how will I get all my chores done before they get back?'

'I've got clinic at two o'clock but I'll help you for an hour. They'll never know,' I conspired.

After clinic I telephoned Chris Jentry to do my own referral to the Children's Department.

'Can we see her at home to do the paperwork?' he asked.

'That would be difficult. Dr Drake has said we can use his office. Can you see Valerie there instead? Do it all in one go; you have both our referrals.'

'You want her to be present at the meeting?' Chris was surprised.

'Yes, if it will speed things up. It is her and her baby's future we're discussing.'

'It's not standard practice but I'll put in my request to Maidstone Authority too. I know the chap there. I'll see if he can pop in with his forms as well when we meet at the surgery.'

'Thank you.'

'A doctor, a social worker and a health visitor doing a joint form – that should speed thing up.' I could hear him turning the pages of his diary. 'I could come out to Totley on 18 December?'

'It has to be a Tuesday.'

'Oh really? Why is that?'

I paused. If I told him would it make it better or worse? What did I actually know? She'd never said anything directly and I'd never seen anything. There was no evidence.

'Sarah, why a Tuesday? Does she work because I need to know if she has an income.'

'She doesn't have paid employment but she has to work on the farm for free and care for the baby. She only gets a break on Tuesday mornings.'

'Oh, that sounds a bit exploitative.'

'It is. Another reason apart from the inadequate living conditions I want to get her and the baby out as soon as possible.'

'I could do 11.30 a.m. on Tuesday, 23 December.'

'Perfect.'

'I'll put in a request to social security for a moving-in allowance as well.'

'I think I can rustle up pots and pans and a kettle if you could help me source some furniture. They don't have much. The baby could do with some new clothes, so could Valerie.'

'Sarah, don't get your hopes up anything will be done about this request till after Christmas at either housing or social security.'

'But you'll get onto them on 2 January?' I pressed. 'And if we get everything signed on 23 December we could put it in the post that afternoon?'

'If you insist.'

'Thank you.'

'I'll see you in a couple of weeks. Hold tight till then.'

I counted on my fingers how many days from 2 January it would take to find housing and do the social security paperwork. I was hopeful we could get her out by the end of February. I pictured Valerie in a clean little flat freshly painted, with nice furniture and the heating on, dressed in a new jumper and jeans, cuddling baby Michael on a comfortable sofa. Surely everyone deserved somewhere safe and cosy to live? There must be a flat, one little flat somewhere in Maidstone or Malling for them, surely there was one; somewhere they'd be safe.

\* \* \*

The next morning I knocked at Lisa-Rose Drury's caravan. I'd had the slip from the hospital to say she'd been released. A young man with chestnut-coloured hair and bright blue eyes answered the door.

'Can I help you?' he asked.

'Mr Drury?' I enquired.

'No, my name's Jones,' he replied cautiously.

'I'm Sarah Hill. Lisa-Rose's health visitor. Is she back from hospital?'

The young man grasped my hand. 'Oh, you're the nurse. Thank you so much. I was only messing with you – I'm Job Drury, Fiance's daddy.' He shook my hand. 'She's over in the wagonette with her mammy. Go on now, they'll be glad to see you. They had a bit of a to-do this morning with the medicine the hospital has given Lisa-Rose. I'll take you over,' he said merrily, jumping down from his caravan to hold open the door for me on the old Romany wagon that belonged to Moses and Queenie Dangerfield.

'It's the nurse to see Lisa-Rose,' he called. 'I'll leave you to it – women's business,' he said with a wink.

'Come in, missus,' I heard Lisa-Rose call.

She was lying on a bed trimmed with lace, her leg raised on a stack of yellow velvet cushions. Queenie was seated at a table covered in a richly embroidered crimson cloth, with a faded plum-coloured fringe, a well-thumbed deck of cards spread out in front of her.

'The cards told me we'd be seeing you today, missus,' cried Queenie.

'The cards?'

'Tarot cards – they belonged to my grandmother. I used to hide under this very table as a child when she did her readings with her crystal ball. Though the caravan came from Moses' people, the furniture is all mine.'

'Sit down, missus,' said Lisa-Rose, tapping the space on the bed beside her. Baby Fiance was loosely swaddled and slumbering next to her mother, her tiny rosebud mouth opening and closing as she dreamt.

'What do you suppose babies dream of?' asked Lisa-Rose.

'Milk and their mothers, I expect,' I ventured.

'Mammy, would you make Fiance up a bottle.'

Queenie rose from her divinations and opened the top cabinet of a wooden dresser painted green and gold. It was stocked to the brim with National Dried Milk.

'I'm glad to be home from that hospital,' said Lisa-Rose with a sigh, shifting herself up in the bed and wincing as she moved her leg.

'The doctors were a bit snooty but the nurses were fine,' added Queenie.

'Oh, yes. Once those gorga nurses find out Mammy tells fortunes all we hear is, "Will this doctor marry me?" "How many charabancs will I have?" Mammy was run off her feet.'

Queenie chuckled. 'I don't mind. It's a gift from God, my girl. We country folk are meant to share it.'

'Love charms. They all want love charms.' Lisa-Rose cast her eye over me. 'Would you like a love charm, missus?'

'On the house,' added Queenie.

I smiled. 'Mr Drury mentioned you'd been having a problem with the medicine the hospital gave you?'

'Oh yes. Job can't bear to see me like this. That's why I'm in here and my dad's bunking down in our caravan. The doctor at the hospital expects me to inject myself with that.' She pointed with a look of disgust to a syringe and small medicine bottle on the bedside table, next to a plastic box for the used syringes. 'It's sadistic.'

'I can't even look at it – makes me feel funny,' said Queenie with a quiver.

I looked at the bottle. 'It's heparin. I could ask the district nurse to come and do it for you.'

Lisa-Rose crinkled her freckled nose. 'Could you do it?'

'I can do it *today*.' Lisa-Rose smiled and let out a sigh and sank back onto her pillows. 'Mrs Dangerfield, may I wash my hands?'

Queenie brought me a beautiful matching ceramic jug and bowl set, a fresh cake of soap and a pristine but threadbare towel. I snapped the top off the vial of heparin and put in the small needle, drawing up the dose and ensuring no bubbles were in it.

'Do you want this in the thigh or the arm?' I asked, syringe at the ready.

'Thigh and then I won't have to look,' replied Lisa-Rose, drawing back the covers and lifting up her white cotton nightgown. She closed her eyes shut tight.

I pinched the flesh of her thigh to inject the fleshy part. 'Take a deep breath for me, and now breathe out, count to five – one, two, three, four and five.' As she did so I gently pushed the needle in – it was over in three seconds. 'Done,' I told her.

'Oh, I barely felt a thing,' remarked Lisa-Rose, examining her thigh. 'Would you do it again tomorrow?'

'I can ask the district nurse to come. But after a few attempts you'll get the hang of it, I'm sure.'

'Oh no, I could never do that. Can't you come instead of the district nurse? We don't like lots of strangers wandering through the camp – there's been enough excitement already.'

'What if I alternate with Nurse Bates?'

'I suppose that will do,' agreed Lisa-Rose with a grin.

Fiance woke and started to cry. Queenie quickly handed her daughter a bottle and the caravan was cosy and quiet once more as she drank the milk in her mother's arms.

'Now give me your hand, missus,' instructed Queenie, taking my palm. She pressed into it, working the flesh with her fingers.

'You're not married. Aren't your hands small? But you've got very flexible fingers, short but flexible. You've got three, no four brothers and sisters. You're going to have an argument with someone high up. Don't let them get you angry or you'll come off the worse for it. Be careful of the stairs – it looks like you're going to have a fall. And there's a man. I see a letter "D". He's from the hills and he's coming towards you on a horse, but he's not sure where he's going. There are two paths in front of him and he doesn't know which to take but you'll help him. You'll spend your life helping people even when you don't want to – it's who you are,' she finished, patting my hands. 'Next time we'll do your horoscope. You tell me your birthday and where you were born and I'll look it up in my ephemeris.'

'All right. For years I thought my birthday was on 22 November and then one day my mother suddenly remembered it was the 23rd. I said to her, "Maybe I was born in the night and you were confused." And my mother replied, "No, I had you after I cleaned the front step in the afternoon."'

'Your mother will live a long life,' she said, looking at my hand once more. 'She'll treasure you in the end.'

# 16

I turned up the volume on the radio as I drove back from Hollow Prospect to my last baby clinic of the year. Karen Carpenter's mellow tones filled my car with a slow rendition of 'Santa Claus Is Coming to Town'. The meeting with Valerie had gone well; it wouldn't be too long now before we'd get her away.

The next record came on: Elvis singing 'Green, Green Grass of Home'. I hadn't even thought about Christmas. It was Christmas Eve tomorrow and I'd made no plans. It'd never mattered if you worked on the wards over Christmas at Hackney. In a hospital there was plenty of fun to be had; I'd always enjoyed it. But Christmas Day was one of the few days of the year health visitors didn't go out. Four days with nothing to do and nowhere to go; I'd catch up on all my jobs and have a Vesta curry in front of *Morecambe & Wise*. There was no point in cooking a turkey for only me.

I pulled up at the clinic and popped back to Ivy Cottage to collect my parcels. Flo and I had spent the entire previous evening wrapping presents for the children and labelling them with age-appropriate stickers so we'd know whether a gift was suitable for a girl under one or a boy aged three. Hermione, Mrs King and I had been stockpiling gifts for weeks and getting donations from local businesses to eke it out. We'd all spent the weekend baking mince pies, and I tried out a new gingerbread recipe to make a little gingerbread house; I suppose a lack of bright lights on the weekend did make for developing your culinary skills. I'd been taken aback when all the volunteers had agreed to dress up for the party; Hermione had told me that usually all the grannies and aunties turned up as well as the mums and babies for the clinic Christmas party. Forewarned, I arrived with bin bags full of gifts just in time for doors opening.

Miss Elena was up a stepladder hanging paper chains, while Mrs Bunyard was telling her it wasn't straight. They'd even wrapped the scales in golden tinsel.

'Not very traditional,' Hermione said, noting the bin bags. 'Here, give them to me. I found a lovely red sack in the dressing-up box at the village hall. Now, let me introduce you to Father Christmas.'

'Ho, ho, ho,' he called. Mr King had been volunteered to play Saint Nicholas and was already in situ on a tinsel-covered chair. 'And have you been a good girl this year?' he said with a chuckle.

'I'll be your helper today, Father Christmas,' said Hermione. 'I'm the Sugar Plum Fairy,' she announced with relish, and with her usual dramatic flourish produced a silver and lilac wand and a pair of fairy wings out of nowhere.

'Oh, Miss Drummond, that's marvellous.'

Hermione grinned. 'Places, everyone. Mrs King, if you would.'

Mrs King put on a red Santa hat and began to play 'We Wish You a Merry Christmas' on an upright piano.

'Where did you get the piano?' I asked.

'We wheeled it over from the village hall at lunchtime,' Mr King informed me. 'It nearly gave me a hernia.'

'Pish-posh,' chastised Hermione. 'The doors, Miss Hill, if you please.'

With huge excitement I threw open the clinic doors and it felt like half of Totley had come to join in the fun. In between weighing babies and the usual consultations we served mince pies and cups of tea, gave every child a gift and sang carols round the piano. The time simply flew by. I clocked Mrs Bunyard knocking back the sherry in the corner with her pals. She caught my eye and called, 'Your very good health, Nurse.'

By four o'clock the clinic was a happy mess of shredded wrapping paper, crumbs, spilt drinks and decimated strings of tinsel.

'You ladies leave this up to me,' instructed Flo.

'Absolutely not,' replied Mrs King. 'If we all pitch in we'll have it cleaned up in no time.'

We locked the doors and got to work, singing as we cleaned up. It finally felt like I belonged in Totley. It had been so much effort preparing everything but seeing all those happy children was completely worth it.

'What are you doing for Christmas, Sarah?' asked Hermione as we swept.

'Nothing,' I answered.

'Not anything?' she said, gasping. I nodded. 'Why ever not?'

'I've been so busy I forgot to make any arrangements.'

'What are we going to do with you? You'll come to me for Christmas Day lunch, won't you?'

'That's very kind of you, Hermione. I wouldn't want to impose.'

'I insist. Come back with me after the morning service. It'll be just me and Etty.'

'Thank you. I'd love to.'

'Well, I think we've all earned a festive tipple,' announced Mrs King.

'I should say so,' cheered Hermione.

There was a knocking at the doors. I unbolted them. It was Alan Bunyard.

'I'm afraid you've missed the clinic Christmas party, Mr Bunyard,' I told him.

'It's not that, Nurse. Susie needs to see you right away. Will you come?'

'Of course, I'll get my coat and bag.'

'Thank you, Nurse. I'll head back and tell her you're coming.'

'What's happened?'

'Susie will want to tell you herself. We'll see you in a bit,' he confirmed, racing off into the twilight.

The Bunyards' door was freshly painted. No more peeling paint but a smart yellow front door decorated with a Christmas wreath we'd made in the Mother's Interest Group. Alan Bunyard opened the door.

'Thank you for coming, Nurse.'

I followed him through to the sitting room. Susan was on the sofa and next to her was a small blonde girl with blue ribbons tied in each curly bunch of fine hair, dressed in a short blue smock with cream puffed sleeves and a frilly petticoat. In her small arms she was cradling baby Sharon as she sat hip to hip with Susan Bunyard on their sofa. Susan looked up at me, tears in her eyes.

'Miss Hill, I'd like you to meet someone very special. This is Michelle, my little girl,' she told me, throwing her arms around the child and hugging her close.

'Hello. Are you a friend of my mummy's?' asked Michelle.

I bobbed down to face her. 'I am,' I answered. I felt a lump in my throat at the sight of her. 'And I'm so very happy to meet you, Michelle. Your Mummy talks about you all the time.'

Michelle smiled. 'This is my baby sister,' she told me.

'Yes, and you're holding her beautifully, you clever girl.'

'Would you like a mince pie and some milk, Michelle?' asked her mother.

'Oh, yes,' she answered.

'Here, give the baby to …' her voice tailed off as she met her husband's eyes.

'Daddy,' suggested Alan Bunyard, taking the baby and sitting next to Michelle on the sofa. 'Shall we watch *Jackanory*?' he asked her, switching on the television. 'I do like a bit of Jane Asher,' he commented.

'Do you now?' said Susan, her hands on her hips as she paused in the doorway to the kitchen. 'Come with me, Nurse.'

'How is Michelle here?' I asked in a whisper.

Susan Bunyard was bouncing with excitement. 'Didn't the Children's Department phone you?'

'I've not been in the office all day.'

'We got a phone call early this morning. Aunty Mildred had a myo-something fraction.'

'A myocardial infarction?'

'That's the one,' she said, pouring out milk into a beaker and putting mince pies onto a tray. 'We raced to see her in hospital and when we got there a social worker was with Michelle. Apparently Aunty had got terrible chest pains in the night but managed to call an ambulance before she collapsed, and it's not the first time by all accounts.'

'How is she now?'

'It doesn't look good, poor Aunty. I felt so sorry for her when I saw her in the hospital bed. Anyway, it made her realise she can't go on pretending she's Michelle's mother. The child knows she's not. We've only had a few visits but there's a bond between us, I know there is.'

'So, Michelle's going to be living with you?'

'Yes. The social workers said they'd usually try and place a child with a relative in these circumstances. It's not official yet but she's mine. I've got my baby back,' she cried with joy. 'It's the best

Christmas present in the whole wide world. I'm so lucky, I'm so happy – I don't deserve it.'

'Yes, you do,' I insisted.

'We're going to be a proper family. Our first Christmas and it's going to be the best ever. It's like a fairy story,' she added as we returned to Alan, Michelle and Sharon snuggled up watching *Jackanory*.

Susan snuggled in with them and I drank in their happy scene and thanked God. I couldn't have wished for more.

Christmas Eve and it was snowing. Not beautiful big flurries but sleet that showered down and made the roads slippery and treacherous. Poor Laura's car was already in the garage after she'd gone into a ditch at the beginning of the week. I didn't fancy driving back through the winding country lanes in the dark. I glanced down at my clock on the icy dashboard – it was only 1.30 p.m., so plenty of time to see Mrs Seaton and get back to Totley before nightfall, I thought. When the shower stopped a mist crept over the hills and I had to use my fog lights to see the road ahead. As my Mini attempted the ascent to Homestead Farm it started to skid. I could see the farmhouse over the fields and decided to pull into a passing space and make the rest of the way on foot.

Crossing the fields, I could see a man on horseback thundering across the open countryside; within minutes he was upon me as I climbed over a stile to the Seatons' land. The rider jumped the fence, showering me with cold muddy water as his horse's hooves hit the ground.

'What do you think you're playing at?' I shouted at him. My skirt and coat were drenched with dirty water. But he didn't look back. Steaming, I marched on. As I got near the farmhouse I saw him letting his horse drink from a cow trough.

His mount was at least 17 hands and the man cut a towering dark figure in tweeds.

'You did that on purpose,' I scolded him. But he turned his head the other way and refused to even look at me. 'I said you splashed me on purpose. Who do you think you are? What sort of person does that!' Still he continued to fiddle about with the stallion's bridle and fidgeted in the saddle as his horse drank deeply. I noticed an engraving on the saddle, 'Dash'. It must be the horse's name. 'You watch it, I've got my eye on you,' I warned, as incensed I stomped off to the farmhouse. Mrs Seaton was at the door.

'What's happened to you, Nurse?' she called.

'That man splashed me,' I waved wildly in his direction but he'd already galloped off.

'That'll be Captain Beauchamp-Smith. The New Year's Day hunt passes this way. He'll be ensuring his horse knows the course,' Mrs Seaton concluded. 'Master of Foxhounds, he is.'

I bit my lip; it wasn't professional to start banging on about that stupid man and stupid hunting. God, he was rude. He wouldn't even look at me. Mr Flaming High and Mighty. I remembered Queenie and her prediction – oh, just my luck.

Shaking off my mood I turned on my brightest smile. 'Mrs Seaton, you said on the telephone you were worried about some marks on the baby's body?'

'Yes, follow me, Nurse. Tim's having his nap.'

I softly pulled up the cover to examine baby Tim's legs and arms as he slumbered in the wicker basket and then tucked him back in.

'Nothing to worry about, Mrs Seaton. That criss-cross pattern on his arms and legs is where he's pressed himself up against the sides of the basket. The lines on his ankles are from the ribbing on his socks.'

Mrs Seaton put her hand over her mouth to stop herself laughing. 'Oh dear, Nurse. I'm so sorry to call you out for that.'

'It's not a problem, Mrs Seaton. It happens quite a lot. Anyway, how's your week been?'

'Dreadful. I had hardly any problems feeding Gary, Karen or Tina but Tim's another story. One of my breasts hurt so badly I can hardly bear to put him on. It feels lumpy.'

'Would you like me to take a look?'

'If you would, Nurse.'

She opened her shirt and I examined the breast. 'It does looks swollen,' I confirmed. 'Does it hurt badly when you feed?'

'I dread it. And I'm so busy with the other three, as well as with running the house – and we're shorthanded in the dairy. Some of the cows are in a bad way; the vet's in with them now.'

'Sounds like you're rushed off your feet.'

'I am. And it's Christmas Day tomorrow. I've still got a hundred and one things to do.'

'I think you've got a blocked duct. You'll need to drink lots of fluids. You can try to clear the blockage after giving the baby a really good feed by massaging the breast under warm water. Or an ice pack might help. If you've got some frozen peas I could make you up one if you like to ease it?'

'Please, Nurse. The deep freezer is in the pantry.'

I fetched the frozen peas and put them in a plastic bag, wrapping them in a clean tea towel.

'Here, press down on the breast with this.'

Mrs Seaton slipped in the ice pack. 'Ah, that feels a little better. I am worried he's not getting enough milk though. He gets so cross with me when I feed him. I think he doesn't like me sometimes.'

'That's not true. You're everything to him. Most babies get a bit hot and bothered during feeding. How many wet and dirty nappies are you getting at the moment?'

'Not many the last few days and the last one he did was a funny colour.'

'Can I take a look?'

'Help yourself, Nurse,' she instructed, waving at a pail in the corner filled with terry-towelling nappies. 'I haven't had a chance to put a wash on today yet.'

The nappy contained only a tiny bit of light-green poo that stained the nappy. It was a hunger stool. I sat in the armchair opposite Mrs Seaton.

'Tim's a rather long baby. They are often more challenging to feed.'

'Are they, Nurse?'

'Sometimes. How much are you getting to eat and drink yourself, Mrs Seaton?'

'I'm lucky if I grab myself a piece of toast and a cup of coffee.'

'It must be very hard.'

'It is, Nurse,' she answered slightly tearfully. 'He's not getting enough, is he? I knew it, really. I can just about stand it for seven minutes and then I have to take him off.'

'We can sort this out together. First of all I'm going to go to the kitchen and get you something. You can't take care of your family if you don't have a bit of time to look after yourself. Eating and drinking is essential. Let's look at latching and treating the breast so it's more comfortable for both of you. Before and after you feed, try rubbing the nipple with some breast milk. It can be quite soothing and make the latch more comfortable. With a bit of luck you could both be as right as rain in a few days.'

'Do you think so, Nurse?'

'I do. When Tim wakes up would you like me to look at how he's latching so we can check you're as comfortable as possible?'

'That sounds like a plan to me, Nurse. It's been a few years since I did it with Karen. I had the other children one after another but Tim's a late entry.'

Once Mrs Seaton was feeding comfortably I went to the kitchen to make her a drink and a snack.

'Where are the other children?' I asked.

'In the parlour. They're on their father's heels today.'

'Keen farmers?'

'No, the cat had kittens. She's a secretive madam; she went missing at the end of September and then we found her in the dairy this morning with three of them running around. Phil's put them in a sack and said he'll drown them as soon as the vet's gone.'

'Oh dear.'

'I know, but I don't have the energy to argue with him. We're overrun with cats as it is – there's too many mouths to feed already. If the kids can't find homes for them by teatime it'll be curtains for those poor little kittens.'

'How many kittens did you say there were?'

'Three.'

'I'll take them. I'm sure I can find homes for them.'

'You are tender, Nurse. You'd never make a farmer's wife. I'll take you to the parlour once Tim's finished his feed.'

I accompanied Mrs Seaton to see the herd. Mr Seaton was having a moan to the vet as he examined several of the cows. I couldn't see the vet at all – he was only a pair of dark green wellies poking out from behind a Friesian, a pair of rubber gloves on an udder as the cow bellowed at his touch.

'It may be raining today but the water shortage this year has just about finished us off,' moaned Mr Seaton. 'And now the government says they're going to ban irrigation. I'd like them to tell me what to feed the cows. Cattle's practically eaten all the silage we made this year already and there's no cud for them; fields are practically bald. We're using the emergency clamps already – I've a hundred pedigree Friesian milkers and no grass, no kale and very little choice but to buy it in. Where's the profit in that?' the farmer continued. 'Take Hill Cott Farm. I heard they lost £6,000 on summer milk production alone. We're all having to feed in bought-in barely straw; £30 a tonne and we're already on the concentrates. If this water shortage goes on I reckon we'll have to sell off some of the beef cattle early. Food prices go up and who does the government blame – us farmers. But it's not us who pockets the money – we're only trying not to make a loss.'

'How far before calving did you dry off the cows, Mr Seaton?' the vet asked, pulling off his rubber gloves as he emerged from behind a cow. He was in his early thirties, dressed in brown overalls over a thick green bobbly jumper and jeans. I recognised that familiar Scottish accent from my childhood. He pushed his long auburn fringe out of his green eyes, not realising an audience had gathered during the examination. I took my place with Mrs Seaton holding baby Tim and the three other Seaton children to lean against the gate of the pen waiting to hear the vet's diagnosis.

'I gave them a couple of weeks,' Mr Seaton answered grouchily.

'Have you noticed any clotting in the milk?'

He shrugged. 'A bit.'

'Have they been off their food?'

'Bit,' mumbled Mr Seaton.

'Oh, Phil,' scolded Mrs Seaton. 'Is it mastitis, Veterinary?'

'It is. One quarter of the udder is red and inflamed on most of them but on a couple it's more. The affected cows are in a lot of pain.'

'I know how they feel,' said Mrs Seaton.

The vet's cheeks went pink. He looked away, embarrassed, and returned to the cattle. 'They'll need clean dry bedding and you'll need to keep their udders clean and dry too. Keep the affected cows separated from the rest of the herd until it clears and I recommend a teat dip after milking. I'm prescribing inframammary administration of antibiotics. It'll be one tube per quarter and ensure the parlour is thoroughly clean after each milking,' instructed the vet, now packing away his things.

'Don't you worry, he will,' confirmed Mrs Seaton. 'Phil, I've got a new baby to take care of, for heaven's sake, and the kids. You can't look after the herd for a few weeks on your own without letting standards slip. After all the work we've put into these animals.'

'You know how short-handed we've been, Lynda,' whined Mr Seaton. 'I don't have the same way with the cows as you. They miss you, love. So do I.'

Mrs Seaton turned her back on him. 'Kids, your father won't be drowning any kittens.'

'Now hang on a minute, Lynda.'

'What's this, Mr Seaton?' interrupted the vet.

'Nothing, nothing,' dismissed the reprimanded dairy farmer.

'The nurse said she'd take the kittens and find them homes.'

Suddenly six pairs of eyes were on me. I shifted uncomfortably.

'That's very kind of you, Nurse,' said Mr Seaton, and he thrust a sack full of kittens into my arms. The bag was a mass of kicks and mewls – I didn't fancy carrying it across the fields to my Mini.

'I've got a cat carrier you can borrow in the back of my Land Rover,' offered the vet shyly.

'Thank you. Well, merry Christmas,' I wished the Seaton family. It was getting dark and I was eager to get back to my car.

I followed the vet to his mud-splattered Land Rover parked in the farmyard.

'It's very nice of you to take in the kittens,' he told me as he rooted out a carrier from the back of the car.

'I've been thinking of getting a cat, so I'll only need to find homes for two.'

'May I?' He smiled and I gladly passed him the sack. He reached in and pulled each little ball of fur out by the scruff of its neck and gently placed it in the carrier. First came a little ginger one, then two black and whites.

'Which one do you think you'll keep?'

'I like the look of the ginger one. Is it a she or a he?'

'You're a nurse,' he teased.

'I didn't get a very good look and I was poorly the day we covered feline anatomy in preliminary training school.'

He smiled. 'She's a female. The other two are males.'

'Perfect.'

'I can pop over and give them a check and their immunisations if you like?' I was taken by surprise. 'Free of charge, of course,' he added.

'That's very kind of you.'

'It's nothing,' he dismissed, tousling his hair and opening the car door.

'Can I give you a lift?'

'My Mini's parked nearby,' I replied, starting to head towards the stile – it was starting to get dark.

'You didn't tell me your name or where you live.'

'I'm Sarah Hill. I'm at Ivy Cottage on the Main Road in Totley.'

'Danny Rennie. Shall I come over on Boxing Day?'

'You're working on Boxing Day?'

'I wondered if you'd like to go for a drink,' he invited. A little gathering of Seatons had gathered to watch. Danny the vet's cheeks pinked once more.

'All right. Pick me up at six o'clock.'

'You're a dark horse, Veterinary!' shouted Mr Seaton.

Danny jumped into his Land Rover and sped off. I didn't like being asked out in front of clients but by the looks of it Danny was mortified.

Somehow I'd gone from the prospect of being alone in my flat over Christmas to having a lunch invitation at Hermione's, a date on Boxing Day and three lively kittens to keep me company over the break. It was almost dark when I reached my Mini. I put the kittens into the boot and turned on the engine, eager to be home, but the engine was dead. Oh no! I'd stupidly left my fog lights on. I'd been two hours at Homestead Farm. I pressed my forehead against my hands on the steering wheel and exhaled, trying to regain my composure. I didn't fancy trekking across the fields in the dark back to the farm. I remembered there was a red phone box about a quarter of mile down the road so set off with my torch to see if by some miracle Trev Bowyer was still working on Christmas Eve at Totley Garage. I sat and waited, wrapping a blanket round me and snuggling with the kittens for warmth. It started to sleet again.

Bless Trev, he was only 20 minutes and he got my little Mini started in no time. I asked him how much I owed him. He insisted, 'No charge, Nurse. It's Christmas.' I learned that day that patience and perseverance are what mums and newly qualified health visitors need to get them through.

I was glad to get home to the peace and tranquillity of Ivy Cottage. My new flatmates proved to be a bit of a handful at first as they darted straight out of the cat carrier and under the sofa. I made a basket for them out of an old vegetable box and lined it with a dark orange jumper I'd been unsuccessfully attempting to knit. It was too holey to wear but made a perfect kitten comforter.

Little by little I tempted each kitten out with a saucer of milk and tiny bits of chicken from the pot-roasted old hen I was cooking. Flo had given me a hen the day before and it would last for the next week; just as well as I'd not had time to do any shopping. After their near-death experience the three little kittens were soon fast asleep and I ate my dinner on my lap in front of the telly. Afterwards I poured a generous measure of port and lemonade and snuggled up on the sofa to watch *The Old Grey Whistle Test*.

It was comforting to lift the sleeping ginger kitten out of the box and stroke her soft fur as she curled up on my lap and purred melodically. 'I think I'll call you Ginger, puss,' I told her.

Queen were performing at the Hammersmith Odeon. I'd buy myself a record of 'Bohemian Rhapsody' as a Christmas present, I decided, nodding along to the music. Who needed the bright lights of London when you could enjoy Freddie Mercury from the comfort of your own home? This was my real life, and it was a good life.

## 17

First day of a New Year and where was I? Casualty, that's where. I'd had to wait for hours to get an X-ray and it was only a sprain. Danny could have dressed it himself; he was a vet and there's not much difference, is there? I shouldn't have blamed him; it wasn't really his fault, I suppose. As I waited to be discharged, I thought back over Christmas and remembered with fondness lunch at Hermione's.

I'd been astounded to find that she'd laid the table with a gold-plated silver dinner service, the best Staffordshire dishes and Edinburgh Crystal glasses. It was very grand in her comfortable dining room at River Cottage. The Georgian property had double-fronted bow windows that overlooked the River Walk. You could hear the whooshing of the River Medway as it flowed below us. Spotless cranberry glass pieces lined the window, giving the room a lovely warm feel like a rose-gold-coloured winter sunset. Hermione had swiftly laid another place at the fine mahogany dining table for a member of the congregation we'd discovered was alone on Christmas Day.

I hadn't been going to St Agatha's with the same regularity since Nick's engagement to Felicity Bourne. I watched the nepotistic nativity adorations unfold: Mr Bourne read with solemnity from the Gospel while his sister came to the altar in a very fine hat with a halo-like quality to place the infant Jesus in his cradle. Nick's fiancée was triumphant, prematurely taking on the role of the rector's wife at the church doors. Miss Bourne clutched Nick's arm tightly as they wished churchgoers a Merry Christmas, letting her engagement ring catch the light to dazzle us all.

In the churchyard Mr Hopkins tipped his hat and wished Hermione and I joy, and we discovered that he had planned to stay with his sister in Salisbury for Christmas but the whole family had come down with a bug two days ago and he'd been advised to stay away. Hermione insisted he join us at River Cottage. I watched her tenderly lay his place, gently creasing the folds of the linen napkin to stand to attention and polishing the silver candelabra until it shone. She placed a fine crimson poinsettia on the table and stroked its leaves.

'Did you know the Victorians used to communicate using flowers?' Hermione asked me.

'Did they?

'Oh yes,' my friend replied, reaching for an old book from the shelf and passing it to me. It was beautifully illustrated in watercolours and contained alphabetical lists of flora and fauna written in an elegant hand.

'That was my grandmother's,' Hermione said, beaming with pride. 'So much couldn't be said. So those inscrutable Victorians found ways of using flowers to express their feelings and intentions. Look,' she directed me, pointing to a description in the book. 'Canterbury Bell means "Your letter received". Must have been quite a thrill. Can't you just picture a debutante in her white gown clutching her bouquet, waiting to catch a glimpse of her beau?' Hermione was quite the romantic.

'Such intrigue,' she continued. 'They used gems as well. This brooch belonged to my grandmother,' she said, touching the lapel of her red tunic dress. 'Each gem spells out an acrostic message. This was given to my grandmother before she was married and not by my grandfather either,' she confided with a theatrical wink. 'A gift from a secret love.' Hermione pointed out each gem with her polished index finger. 'You see it has a ruby, emerald, garnet, amethyst, another ruby and a diamond – Sarah, what does that spell?'

'R-E-G-A-R-D, regard!'

'That's right. I do think holding someone in high regard is the most long-lasting kind of love. Look at Mr and Mrs King: a couple who hold each other in the highest of regard.'

'That's really rather lovely,' I replied, leafing through the book. There was a knock on the door.

'Aha, Mr Hopkins! Just in time too – the turkey needs to come out of the oven to rest,' said Hermione, bustling around. She shortly reappeared, followed by Mr Hopkins carrying a bunch of red carnations wrapped in green tissue paper. Hermione immediately arranged them in a cranberry glass vase. I looked up the meaning of red carnations in the Victorian flower book – 'My heart aches for you' – and a flurry of excitement for Hermione and Mr Hopkins ran through me. Could it be a coincidence or had I stumbled upon a drawn-out secret courtship? Why would it need to be secret? After all, they were both unattached mature people.

Hermione's aged mother Etty, who had been having a lie-down, shuffled in bent over her walking stick and joined us for the festive feast. I thought to myself: Oh I see, Hermione isn't free, she isn't free at all.

'You remember Miss Hill and Mr Hopkins, don't you, Etty, dear?' prompted Hermione as we took our seats at the Christmas table.

Etty reached over and snapped off some sticks of celery in a glass jar.

'Yes, of course,' Etty replied in a fine Edinburgh accent and began to munch loudly.

'I hope you don't mind but I've left the leaves on the celery,' explained Hermione, taking a piece. 'They were my favourite part as a child and I used to beg Mother not to throw them away but leave them for me. Do help yourselves. I know celery, crackers and grapes should come at the end of the meal but they are Etty's favourite and she tends to nod off well before dessert. We've rather got into the habit of serving the other way round,' said Hermione with a titter. 'Don't fill up on it though. I've prepared roast turkey with all the trimmings and we've Christmas pudding, mince pies and coffee to get through.'

'It's a very fine spread, Miss Drummond,' praised Mr Hopkins.

'Thank you. I always sit down to a properly laid table even if I'm alone. I think you enjoy the food more.'

I felt slightly ashamed of my previous night in front of the telly.

'Heavens, I forgot the champagne,' exclaimed Hermione, jumping out of her seat. Shortly she returned with beautiful crystal flutes filled to the brim with bubbles and handed them out.

'To the chef,' toasted Mr Hopkins.

'Well, isn't this one of life's lovely moments,' declared Hermione as we chinked glasses.

'And are you still at school?' Etty asked me.

Did she think I was the teacher? 'Mr Hopkins is the headmaster at St Agatha's Primary School,' I answered.

'Yes, I know that,' said Etty patiently. 'But are you still at school?'

'No,' I answered.

'Miss Hill is a health visitor with me at the clinic, Etty dear,' interjected Hermione.

'That's a very big responsibility for a girl,' cautioned Etty.

Yes, I suppose it was really. Etty Drummond had a point. She stayed for the first course of prawn cocktail but after a few mouthfuls of roast turkey announced she was 'done in' and retired to her room for the rest of the evening.

241

At seven o'clock I slipped away too, eager to watch *The Morecambe and Wise Christmas Show* back at Ivy Cottage with Ginger and the other kittens – I didn't want to leave them on their own any longer. Eric Morecambe not only had the same first name as my wonderful dad but looked like him too – it was not to be missed. I kissed Hermione goodbye and thanked her for a wonderful day. As I crunched down the path of the River Walk the sultry tones of Doris Day singing 'Perhaps, Perhaps, Perhaps' were on the night air and back at River Cottage two dancing silhouettes appeared in the bow window of the sitting room. Perhaps Hermione and Mr Hopkins had made their minds up to get started. I did hope so.

Over Boxing Day drinks at The Good Intent, Danny the vet had been keen to hear of my equine experience. Our family pony Frisky had been a bad-tempered piebald Welsh cob partial to biting your thumb, bucking you off and stamping on your foot. I must have had one too many vodka and limes when Danny asked me to go riding with him on New Year's Day.

'I don't have a horse,' I told him, trying to wriggle out of it.

'Neither do I, anymore. I ride the livery horses at Totley Stables. I can borrow one for you.'

'I don't know.'

'I'll choose a nice safe mare, I promise,' he reassured me, patting my hand. His auburn fringe really needed cutting, as it made him blink far too much. It was quite endearing.

I don't think I cut a very fine figure when he collected me on horseback from Ivy Cottage. Not having any proper riding togs and the shops being closed over the holidays I'd dug out from my old trunk a hacking jacket that had belonged to my cousin James, which my Aunt Olive had bestowed on me for reasons I could no longer recall. I teamed it with a blue and white checked shirt, cavalry twill trousers and a pair of lace-up pumps. I felt a little silly with my hair in two plaits under the spare riding hat Danny had brought for me as the hunt passed us by.

My eyes alighted on Felicity Bourne in immaculate dark jacket, cream jodhpurs and shiny knee-length riding boots, her fine blonde hair scooped elegantly into a fancy black hairnet. She sat so confidently on a bay hunter as she drank from a stirrup cup and chatted energetically with the Master, the awful Captain Beauchamp-Smith who'd drenched me on Christmas Eve. The hounds were running around the horses' hooves excitedly outside the pub as they waited for the blast of the trumpet to spring into action. Ted the landlord was passing up the cups to the riders with barely a word of thanks and giving treats from his apron pocket to impatient beagles.

'Are you not joining us, Veterinary?' called Captain Beauchamp-Smith as we passed by.

'Not really my scene,' answered Danny coolly. 'Trot on.' He kicked his horse firmly to pick up its stride and mine followed suit, merrily bouncing along the country lanes. Captain Beauchamp-Smith didn't give me a second look – he was either indifferent or didn't recognise me; actually it was probably both.

'You don't like the hunt?' I asked.

'I cannae stand it,' he responded with a grin. 'Half those Hooray Henrys haven't paid their veterinary fees for six months.'

We trotted onwards towards Fairy Hill but the wind had picked up and it became hard to make any conversation over the howling gusts of air.

'I think there's a storm coming,' I said to Danny, pointing at the looming grey clouds.

'You're right – we better get back before we get a soaking. I'm sorry it's not been a better day for it, but I've enjoyed spending time with you, Sarah.'

'Me too, Danny.'

'Another time?' he asked as he turned his horse's head to follow the trail home.

There was a sudden blast of a trumpet and my horse's ears pricked up. In the distance we heard the cry of 'View halloo'.

'Looks like the hounds have picked up the scent of some poor fox,' said Danny shaking his head sadly.

Within moments the hounds and riders came thundering across the field surrounding us. We tried to get to one side and out of the way but my horse started to follow the hunt and ran away with me. Danny galloped after me, trying to get hold of my reins. As we came up to the stile at Homestead Farm I came tumbling off. Fortunately, I was at the back of the pack and didn't get trampled. Danny jumped off his horse.

'Sarah, are you hurt?' he cried, rushing to my aid.

'I don't think so,' I answered, covered in mud and feeling very sore and shaken.

'Here, take my arm,' offered Danny, placing a strong arm around my shoulders. As I pressed my hands on the ground to get up, I felt a rush of pain in my left arm and moaned.

'You *are* hurt. Here, let me see,' sympathised Danny.

'It's only a sprain,' I said. 'Take me home and I can patch it up.'

'No, I'll take you to Casualty and get it X-rayed to be on the safe side.'

'On New Year's Eve – are you mad? Take me home.'

'Doctor's orders, I'm afraid. Come on,' he insisted, hoiking me up to my feet.

'You're a vet,' I protested.

'Do as you're told or I'll put you down,' he warned, his look of concern turning back to that cheeky smile. 'Do you think you could ride back to Totley and then I can drive us to Maidstone?' he asked.

'I'm sure I'll be OK on the nice safe mare you found for me,' I teased. 'We better hurry as it does looks like it's going to blow one heck of a gale.'

Driving back from the hospital with my arm in a sling I thought the Land Rover would turn over as it was a terrible night. When we got back to Totley the village was in darkness, and branches had fallen into the road, making it a treacherous drive. I found some candles under the kitchen sink and attempted to illuminate Ivy Cottage.

'What a day. I hope no one's been hurt in the storm,' I said.

'I don't think it's safe for me to drive back to Malling – I might get struck by lightning,' said Danny, stroking one of the black and white kittens, pulling his ears and tickling him under the chin as the tiny cat nibbled his fingers.

'That's true, I suppose. You can sleep on the sofa.'

'Thank you. I'll make us supper, as you need to rest that arm.'

'We've no light and no power. How do you propose to do that?'

He opened up the kitchen cupboard and rummaged through, shining his candle in to see what delicacies I had in reserve.

'Did I tell you I'm a vegetarian?' His muffled voice echoed from the darkness of the kitchen cupboard.

'No. My best friend from Hackney, Maggie, she's a vegetarian. But I don't see how you'll heat us up baked beans on toast.'

'You're in for a treat, Sarah. Because I've found a packet of breadsticks and an almost full tube of squeezy cheese. Let me prepare you one now. Do you like your cheese spread or piped?'

'Piped, please.'

'*Voilà, Mademoiselle,*' he said, squirting the cheese onto a bread-stick with a flourish. 'Your dinner is served. And for my next trick I'm going to make the red wine disappear from this glass,' he announced, pouring a glass.

'When did you get that bottle?'

'Aha! A magician never reveals his secrets and I never like to come to a home for the first time empty-handed,' he replied, handing me the glass. 'Happy New Year, Sarah.'

'It's almost the second of January.'

'But I'm Scottish. We first-foot until February, I'll have you know.'

'Well, there's a lump of coal in the scuttle you're welcome to.'

'The famous generosity of the English,' he teased and I threw a cushion off the sofa at him. He caught it and knelt down on the floor next to the sofa and placed it back gently.

'We've no telly to watch,' he observed, nodding towards the blank screen. 'Which is a shame because I don't have a TV and it'd be nice to watch something.'

'Well, you'd better do your party piece,' I suggested.

'My party piece?'

'Aye, it'll take my mind off my sore arm.'

Danny cleared his throat and began:

Ae fond kiss, and then we sever;
Ae fareweel, alas, for ever!
Deep in heart-wrung tears I'll pledge thee,
Warring sighs and groans I'll wage thee!
Who shall say that Fortune grieves him
While the star of hope she leaves him?
Me, nae cheerfu' twinkle lights me,
Dark despair around benights me.

I'll ne'er blame my partial fancy;
Naething could resist my Nancy;
For to see her was to love her,
Love but her, and love for ever.

246

Had we never loved sae kindly,
Had we never loved sae blindly,
Never met – or never parted –
We had ne'er been broken-hearted.

'I can't remember the rest,' he mumbled

'That's all right. I don't like Robbie Burns much,' I responded.

He leant in to kiss me but there was a huge flash of lightning followed by a crash. We ran to the windows.

'Oh, my goodness. A tree has fallen into Totley Garage. Quick, bring a torch and my bag. They've got four children in that flat,' I ordered.

We ran out into the storm to see if we could help. Fortunately, Trev and Jackie Bowyer and all the children were unharmed. But the garage was a wreck.

Trev was in despair. 'We're ruined, we're ruined,' he cried, running his hands through his hair.

'It's just a setback, Trev, love,' soothed Jackie. 'It'll take some time but we'll get it all fixed and it'll be up and running in no time.'

'You don't understand. I haven't paid the insurance premium for three months,' he wailed. 'I couldn't spare it after the new baby and Christmas. I'm so sorry, I've failed you all.'

It took three days for the power to come back to Totley. For most of us it meant cooking on camping stoves and doing clinic by candlelight but Totley Garage didn't open again.

# 18

After I cooked us a vegetarian supper Danny and I watched *When the Boat Comes In*, sitting side by side at Ivy Cottage, eyes glued to the box. He yawned and put an arm round my shoulder.

'Isn't this cheery?' he commented.

'Socialist Great Depression stories on the Tyneside? Oh aye, it's a barrel of laughs.'

'You love it.'

'I do. I think it's brilliant. I'm quite taken with James Bolam as Jack Ford.'

'Those Geordies think they're tough but we'd make mince-meat of them in Glasgow.'

I bit my lower lip and looked over his soft hands, freckled pink-cheeked face and long auburn hair – personally, I didn't think he'd last two minutes on Sauchiehall Street on a Saturday night.

'Shall we make this a regular Thursday night thing?' he enquired. 'I make supper and we watch telly?'

'Aye, why not?' he said, stretching out his long legs onto my glass coffee table and crossing them at the ankles. His thick blue socks needed darning; I wasn't going to do it.

'Is it my cooking, my company or my television that you're so keen on?' I ventured.

'Why, it's quite a package, Sarah. I'd find it hard to pick between the three.'

I dug him in the ribs. 'How are you still single?' His face dropped for a moment. 'What is it?' I asked.

'Nothing.' He paused. 'I don't want you to think I've got my feet under the table too quickly.'

'Or on top of the coffee table?'

'How about I take you dancing?'

'What, to Maidstone?'

'Better.' He rubbed his hands with glee.

'A night in London?' I sat up eagerly.

'A ceilidh,' he replied, his grin almost the width of his face.

'Are you asking me to go with you to Scotland, because, Danny ...'

'No, not Scotland – hold your horses there, lassie. I'm a well-respected veterinarian, I've my reputation to think of. No, no, no. I'm inviting you to accompany me to an evening of fine food, conversation and dancing at Totley Grange with the toffs.'

'You're not part of the county set,' I scoffed.

'No, but they are hosting a Burns Night for the Caledonian Society and need a genuine Scot to add authenticity to the proceedings.'

'Robbie Burns again,' I groaned.

'You told me you loved Scottish country dancing.'

'I do. I'm not very keen on dour poetry and haggis.'

'I'll nae have any haggis. We'll have two plates of neeps and tatties and a wee dram to keep out the cold,' he responded, putting on a thick Scottish drawl.

'At Totley Grange?'

'Yes. Lady Cecilia is the President of the Caledonian Society and she's asked me personally to be the Treasurer.'

'The what?'

'It's good for business. Don't look so disappointed. Not all of us are born with a silver spoon and a pony. Some of us have to climb our way up the greasy pole.'

I folded my arms and huffed.

'Oh, come on. You'll enjoy it. A chance to have a wee nosey round the big house,' he said with wide puppy-dog eyes.

'All right,' I agreed reluctantly. Actually, I had a primary visit to do at Totley Grange for one of the staff but I couldn't tell him that.

I loaded up my Mini for a day's visiting. Wellies, torch and now sack cloth and a shovel. I'd got stuck in a snow drift and Danny had explained if you put the cloth under the wheels you can usually dig yourself out and drive off. I didn't want to get caught out in another cold snap. Over the road Trev Bowyer was tidying up the forecourt of the garage and caught my eye.

'I'm getting things shipshape before I head off,' he explained.

'Where are you going, Trev?' I trotted over.

'Hasn't Jackie told you?' I shook my head. 'I've taken a six-month stint as a merchant seaman. If we're careful I can send money home and save up to do the repairs on the garage and be open again by summer.'

'Will you be away the whole time?'

'No, I'll be back every six to eight weeks. You'll not be rid of me that easily, Nurse,' he said with a chuckle.

'When do you set sail?'

'Tomorrow,' he replied, and for a moment all the wind truly went out of his sails.

'Lots of luck, Trev. You'll be home before you know it.'

He gulped and I thought it best to be off before it got emotional, as he wouldn't want that.

'Nurse,' he cried out and came jogging after me as I got into the car. 'Would you keep an eye on my Jackie? I know she acts tough, but it's all front.'

'Of course, I will,' I reassured him.

&#42; &#42; &#42;

Totley Grange had a wonderful view of the village; it was completely unobscured. Mr King had told me there'd been a hamlet once but during the seventeenth century but the incumbents of the big house felt it spoilt the view and had it demolished before tearing down their own manor to build an even grander one.

At the entrance I passed through two concrete pillars with a lodge on either side and followed the drive to the red-brick house. Two lines of conical conifers stood sentry duty on either side of the large expanse of lawn flanked by herbaceous borders and mature shrubs and trees. Even the stables and coach house were rather grand and I noticed a young groom brushing down Dash, Captain Beauchamp-Smith's horse.

It was a large, imposing baroque home with long elegant plinths all along the façade and a good many sash windows. A central glazed door stood at its centre encased by panelled pilasters that hooded the entrance. At the top was a pyramid-shaped clock tower complete with both a bell and a weather-vane.

I pulled the bell and waited and waited, but there was no answer. Eventually, I gave the large door a little push and it creaked open to reveal a fine entrance hall with a black and white marble floor and dark wooden panelling. The staircase was open and mounting clockwise at the west of the hall as it ascended two storeys. I called out but there was still no answer.

I could hear a distant thud and followed it down a passageway to the kitchen. Standing at a huge wooden table was a young Filipino woman with a saw in her hand attempting to carve up a large hand and spring of pork. She had long shiny black hair pulled back in a high ponytail and wore a white apron over a faded black dress with a white Peter Pan collar.

'Mrs Reyes?' I asked.

She stopped and eyed me up. 'Yes,' she replied hesitantly, a slight twitch in her dark eyes and full lips.

'I'm Sarah Hill, the health visitor. I've come to see how you and your new baby are getting along,' I explained.

'Excuse me,' she replied, wiping her hands on her apron and smiling warmly. 'I'm preparing tonight's dinner. Lady Cecilia has a lot of friends coming over.'

'You're working?' I enquired

'Yes, I was straight back to work as soon as I came home from hospital. Lady Cecilia said there is to be as little disruption to the running of the house as possible. I even scrubbed the hall before I went to have Crystal,' she told me.

'You're entitled to six-week maternity leave, you know.'

'No, no. I don't get anything. I'm not British, you see. I'm from the Philippines. We've only worked here three years. We aren't entitled to anything.'

I was about to ask who told her that when Lady Cecilia herself breezed into the kitchen wearing a fur coat and mustard-coloured headscarf. She pulled off her coat and threw it to Mrs Reyes, 'Hang that up, Cristina. Oh, are you the nurse?' she asked with a smile, showing both rows of small white teeth.

'Yes.'

The Lady of the Manor was wearing a red and pink checked skirt suit with a huge flouncy bow in the same material at the neck. She patted her hair back into place as she unpinned the scarf – she rather put me in mind of Princess Margaret.

'I've been to inspect the orchid house,' she told me. 'Cristina, where is José? My *Phalaenopsis* needs much more watering.'

'I'll tell him, Lady Cecilia,' replied Mrs Reyes as she picked up the saw again and tried to make the best of such a cheap cut. Her baby was lying in a wicker basket on the table top amongst cabbages and potatoes. The best silverware lay half-polished – there was so much work to do. Surely Mrs Reyes couldn't be expected to do all this alone and look after a baby?

Lady Cecilia poked her upturned nose into the basket. 'You'll smother that baby by keeping it in this kitchen,' she scolded Mrs Reyes. 'Nurse, I've told Cristina it is normal in England to wrap the baby up and let her sleep under the apple trees in the orchard for a few hours while you get on. I had a January baby and that's what I did on Nanny's day off,' she informed me, confident in her advice.

'Mrs Reyes, is there somewhere I could examine you?' I asked. I knew Ernestine would have checked her over but I wanted a chance to talk to Mrs Reyes away from her overbearing employer.

'Yes, in our room. Follow me.'

'All right. You can have five minutes,' assented Lady Cecilia. 'Then would you bring me tea in the library,' and off she trotted with her immaculate head held high.

Mrs Reyes reached into the basket and gathered up Crystal. 'Follow me, Miss Hill,' she said. We climbed up a flight of narrow backstairs to the cold attic. Mr and Mrs Reyes's room was sparsely furnished and looked like it hadn't been decorated since the Great War. There was no central heating, only a small fireplace.

'It's a little chilly,' I said, rubbing my hands and stamping up and down.

'Lady Cecilia gives us a small amount of coal for the evening,' said Mrs Reyes. Crystal made a little whimpering sound. 'I think she needs another feed,' said Mrs Reyes, unbuttoning her dress.

'Why don't you get into the bed and wrap the blankets around you and have a rest for half an hour,' I suggested.

She jumped into the bed and sighed. I could see she was absolutely exhausted.

'It must take a lot of people to run a big house like this,' I assumed.

'Apart from the stable boy, there's only me and José, my husband. I cook, clean and do all the shopping. He does the gardening and has a uniform to change into when he chauffeurs Lady Cecilia and the Captain.'

'That's a lot of work for two people, especially with a new baby. Have you had no maternity leave?' Mrs Reyes shook her head.

'How much time do you have off during the week?'

'We never have a whole day off, we work every day. But please don't say anything to Lady Cecilia. I don't want us to lose our place. We're trying to save up to go and see my sister in America but £9 each doesn't last very long.'

'£18 a week – I suppose it doesn't.'

'No, no. £17.95 a month between us because we have board and lodging, you see.'

'You're only paid £18 a month!' That's practically slave labour I thought, horrified at such gross exploitation.

'Yes, but we don't like the food here. We end up having to buy noodles and rice ourselves. And we have to pay for our uniforms,' she explained. 'Lady Cecilia likes us to look just so.'

Does she indeed, I thought. It seemed to me like Lady Cecilia liked to have it all her own way. Surely the Beauchamp-Smiths were breaking the law? You couldn't treat people like that.

Friday evening and I was still in the office deep in thought, chewing my pen lid as I puzzled out the week's events. I'd told Hermione about the Reyeses' situation at Totley Grange.

'What are you going to do about it, Hill?' she asked me in a most sister-like manner. That was the problem. I didn't know what I could do. At least we had a date for Valerie Milstead to move into a new little flat in Maidstone. Only two more weeks to go and then Chris Jentry and I had agreed to sneak her out on market day and help her to move in. All correspondence was coming to me at the clinic so we didn't run the risk of Valerie's uncles reading a letter. Nothing was simple though; people's lives were much more complicated than fixing a broken arm or leg. A fractured spirit was probably the hardest to heal. I'd kept my promise to Trev and popped in to see Jackie Bowyer to check on her and baby Gordon. He was doing well – babbling away, holding his head up and smiling – but the same couldn't be said for his mother.

'All week I've felt numb, Nurse,' Jackie told me plainly, all the good cheer gone from her countenance. 'It's like I'm a robot going through the motions. I get the kids food and clean up but all the time I'm thinking, did Trev really go because of the money, or doesn't he love me anymore? It all feels empty without him. I sat there watching the children stuffing themselves this morning at breakfast, and I thought how did I get here? How did I end up with four kids in a pokey flat and no husband to show for it? It turns my stomach. I can't eat or sleep properly. It sets my heart racing to think of him so far away on that big ocean; anything could happen to him.'

I sat with her and listened. She wasn't herself. 'Do you want me to make an appointment for you to see the doctor?' I asked.

'No, there's nothing wrong with me. He'll think I'm mad. I'm a weak, silly woman,' she told me, her voice completely flat as she stared out. 'It's worse at night, when the kids are in bed and I'm all on my own. I don't think we ever spent a night apart since we were married. I've never been on my own; I went straight from my parents' house to here. And outside it's all the same; everyone's lives go on the same, like the storm wasn't life changing, but it ruined the business, it ruined our lives. I may look the same but I don't feel the same. It's all gone wrong, so wrong, and there's nothing anyone can do about that. Not unless you've got a magic wand. You don't have one of those do you, Nurse?' she asked, trying to smile, but her mouth refused to turn up at the corners.

I didn't have a magic wand and I didn't know how I could help. Trev had only been away a few days but the strain of the storm and closing the business had been too much for Jackie. She wasn't herself – I didn't know what to do.

'I'll pop in again soon but ring me if it gets too much. I may not be able to fix it but two heads are better than one,' I offered.

'Don't you worry about me, Nurse, it'll pass. It takes a bit of getting used to,' she told me, and I prayed it would.

Wrapped up in a large tartan shawl I shivered in Danny's Land Rover as we bumped along the snowy track to Totley Grange for the Burns Night celebrations. A Highland band were already playing on a stage in the entrance hall. Danny looked rather debonair in his kilt and black velvet jacket. My mother had sent me up a shot-silk smoky-grey dress and my black lace-up dancing shoes. A member of the Caledonian Society herself, I fondly recalled how beautiful she had looked at all the fancy gatherings she and my father went to when I was a child in the sixties in Argyllshire. I would never be a beauty like my mother.

'I must say, you look bonnie,' complimented Danny as he took me by the arm and steered us through the crush into the dining room. I thought of poor Mrs Reyes – surely they'd have got caterers in, as she couldn't have been expected to cook for nearly a hundred guests single-handed. I didn't catch so much as a glimpse of her all evening; slaving away below stairs no doubt and with a newborn baby as well. It wasn't right – we were all partying away up here; it wasn't right at all. For a moment I felt cross with Danny for bringing me to Totley Grange; the last thing I wanted to be was part of the county set.

My eyes cast about the room for the comfort of familiar faces. First, I noticed Mrs Bourne seated at one of the many round tables. She was practically full-term, and looked completely fed up in a long emerald green velvet evening gown. Her husband was hosting a table of mainly academic-looking men, staying with them for the weekend perhaps. Rather out of place with these smug balding professors was a young redheaded girl in a tight lavender maxi dress. It was low-cut and her hair was piled high in luscious big curls on top of her head.

'Gosh, who's that?' said Danny with his tongue slightly hanging out as he followed my gaze to the Bournes' table.

'How should I know?' I snapped.

Danny looked a little confused and hurt. I tried to catch Mrs Bourne's eye but she had a glassy look and was staring blankly at the wallpaper. Not much fun for her coming out on a night like this; she couldn't drink, couldn't dance and could go into labour anytime now. The table next to them looked much merrier. Mr and Mrs King and Hermione and Mr Hopkins were enjoying a bottle of wine. Hermione was waving at us. 'Hurry up. I've had to guard the last seats on our table with my life,' she declared. 'They're going to pipe in the haggis any moment now,' she told us excitedly.

Sure enough the bagpipes started and Captain Beauchamp-Smith followed the piper with a haggis destined for the top table and gave the address. Ernestine Higgins and her husband Bob rushed over to join us. 'Sorry we're late,' she whispered.

Bob was in his police dress uniform with several medals on ribbons hanging on his chest. 'What are the medals for?' I asked him.

'I was in the army before I joined the police,' he explained.

'Where were you?'

'Northern Ireland mainly,' he replied and I didn't ask any more questions.

'We were in Germany for a time,' Ernestine added chirpily.

'How was that?' I asked.

'Wonderful. We had a lovely flat and it was good fun on the base. But when Cecily was due to start school we wanted to come home. We bought Bob out of the army and he joined Maidstone Constabulary.'

'Is army life similar to police life?' I enquired.

'I thought it would be a better life,' answered Bob and we let the subject drop. The Higgins were such a cheerful couple but I'd inadvertently touched a nerve.

When they brought round the haggis I picked at my plate and so did Danny.

'What do you think of tonight's fare, lassie?' asked my date.

'I'd have preferred a bowl of leek and potato soup and a bread roll,' I whispered.

'Aye, so would I,' he replied discreetly trying to hide his uneaten food in a paper napkin.

'That's the Chief Constable next to Lady Cecilia,' Bob Higgins told me, pointing at the top table, back to his merry self after a few glasses of vino.

'Trying to get in his good books, are you?' I teased.

'He wouldn't know a mere country constable like me was alive,' replied Bob. 'He's a one for turning up a trouser leg and funny handshakes, if you know what I mean,' he added with a wink as his boss lifted his glass to toast the Queen and the Royal Family.

I was so hungry. It all looked lavish but the food itself wasn't up to much so when the coffee came with pieces of tablet the sudden rush of sugar left me feeling a little queasy and I only half-listened to the songs, recitations and toasts that seemed to go on for hours. Eventually, they finished and the ceilidh started.

'Oh, I do so love to dance,' cried Ernestine, grabbing Bob's hand as the caller announced we take our partners for the Dashing White Sergeant.

'Shall we?' invited Danny.

'I'll hang on for the Gay Gordons,' I replied with a smile, but I couldn't stop myself tapping my feet in time to the music – the highland band were great.

Danny was surprised when Lady Cecilia herself asked him to take a turn around the floor with her and he could hardly refuse. Being alone gave me the opportunity to check on Mrs Bourne, who didn't seem quite right. Mr Bourne had abandoned his pregnant wife to Strip the Willow with the sultry redhead.

'May I join you for a moment?' I asked Mrs Bourne.

'I didn't know you were here, Nurse. Please do,' she invited. 'Sorry, Peter says I'm a bit of a fuzzyhead these days.'

'That doesn't sound like you.'

'It all got a bit too much for me over Christmas. I went to see Dr Botten and he gave me some pills to take if I start to feel,' she paused, searching for a word, 'muddled,' she concluded.

'Do you feel muddled?'

'No, not really. But Peter thinks I get over-emotional. It's funny, I never felt that way when I was pregnant with Antonia or Lizzie. Peter's hopeful it means he'll get a boy this time. Us poor girls, so dispensable,' she concluded, her eyes drifting back to her husband and the redhead.

'Who is she?' I asked.

'A student. Writing a thesis about Kent and the Reformation apparently. Peter thought this would provide some local colour. Can't say I give two hoots for it myself, it's a lot of greedy men with their hands in the honeypot. History would be much more interesting if we knew what the wives and daughters or mistresses even of great men made of it all.'

'Did you meet Mr Bourne at university?' I asked her.

'Lord, no. I met him at a party. I worked in fashion. I used to write for *Vogue* and *Vanity Fair* before my life was all him, and the house and the children. You never realise it was the time of your life until it's gone.'

I was stumped for what to say but Danny came to claim me for the Gay Gordons. He held my waist tightly as we polkaed around the room before taking to the floor with the rest of our party for an Eightsome Reel. A group of police formed the circle next to us as we sped around in a ring. Hermione was the first to do a jig in the centre. Ernestine was the best dancer of us all, but as she pranced around her partner she accidentally bumped into a police sergeant in the next eightsome.

'We're not in the jungle now,' the policeman snapped at Ernestine.

Bob marched up to him, bristling. 'Apologise to my wife, now,' he demanded.

'Watch your mouth, Higgins, or I'll have you on report,' sneered the sergeant.

'Leave it, Bob,' said Ernestine, softly touching her husband's arm.

'Do as your coon wife says,' taunted the sergeant.

Bob raised his hand but Mr Hopkins came between them. 'That's enough. There are ladies present. Mrs Higgins, if you'd partner me, I'd be most obliged.' He offered Ernestine his arm and started the dancing again. At the end of the dance a pink-cheeked Mr Hopkins bowed low and we all curtseyed. The band started another tune. Mr Hopkins fell to his knees, clutching his chest.

'Dylan, what's wrong?' gasped Hermione.

'I think I might be having a heart attack,' answered Mr Hopkins in short breaths.

'Danny, would you call an ambulance please,' I asked, putting Mr Hopkins into the recovery position on the floor as my date ran to find a telephone. Hermione put her shawl underneath Dylan Hopkins's head and stroked his hair as he rested in her lap.

'Try and relax, you wonderful man,' Hermione whispered. 'You're going to be fine. Deep breaths.'

'Will you stay with me, Hermione?' he asked, clutching her hand.

'Always,' replied my elegant friend and somehow the whole room seemed to slip away as I watched the two of them bravely waiting to see how things would turn out.

Danny and I followed the ambulance to the hospital in the Land Rover and waited with Hermione while Mr Hopkins had an ECG. The doctor didn't beat about the bush in his diagnosis.

'You've not had a heart attack, Mr Hopkins.' We all heaved a huge sigh of relief. 'But you are extremely anaemic and your blood pressure is far too high. You must have a minimum of six weeks' rest,' the doctor ordered. 'Or next time you won't be so lucky.'

'That's impossible. I can't be off school for six weeks,' protested Mr Hopkins as he attempted to sit up in bed to argue with the doctor.

Hermione pushed him back on his pillows firmly but gently. 'Yes, you can. And I will be round every day to ensure you do. And you'll find I'm a very strict nurse,' she informed him.

As we drove back to Totley after an eventful Sunday evening Danny remarked, 'Lucky Mr Hopkins, having Hermione to home nurse him for six weeks. Do you still have your nurse's uniform by any chance, Sarah?'

'Why?' I asked.

'I thought I might borrow it for a fancy-dress party,' he replied with a grin. 'Do you have a pair of black stockings to go with it?'

# 19

'Blast it. I've missed half of it,' I complained, pulling off my hat, coat and scarf and throwing them onto the kitchen chair. Danny had been making a pot of vegetable stew on my stove, watching *When the Boat Comes In*, while I taught slings and bandaging to the Malling District Girl Guides in their freezing cold hut. In her capacity as Guides District Commissioner Miss Presnell had volunteered me to teach a weekly first-aid class to pre-adolescent girls for the next six weeks. They met on Thursday evenings from six till eight, making me miss the first bit of our favourite show.

'Sit down, eat your dinner. You haven't missed much,' said Danny, as he dished out the bland-looking soup. I must have wrinkled my nose slightly at the gloopy mixture as he added, 'It's not much, but it's hot.'

'Thank you. It looks very tasty,' I lied. 'What's happened so far?'

'They're all on strike. Coalmen with no coal. Now shush or you'll miss it, and eat your soup,' he told me. 'And don't slurp,' he added with a grin. I very nearly threw my bread roll at him.

When the nine o'clock news came on we switched off the telly and adjourned to the kitchen. Now feeling warmed through and relaxed it was a little bit of domestic bliss as I washed up and Danny dried the dishes. Abba's 'SOS' played softly on the radio in the background.

'Sarah, I've been meaning to tell you something, only I never knew when or how to tell you …' Danny failed to finish the sentence, his voice fading away.

I stopped washing for a moment and gripped the slippery plate in my hands under the water. 'You're not married, are you?' I asked, half laughing and half gasping.

'No, I'm not married,' he replied and turned off the radio.

'Thank heavens for that,' I exhaled and put the last plate on the draining board.

Danny dried his hands on the red-checked tea towel. 'But I am divorced,' he said, sinking into a kitchen chair.

'Oh, I see.' I remained standing, pressing my back against the kitchen sink for support. There's was more to come, I could feel it.

'And I've got two boys.'

'And you never said?'

'No, I don't like talking about it.'

'Why?'

'I'm not ashamed of them. They're fine boys. It's me and their mother I'm ashamed of, we've made such a mess of things.'

'What are their names?'

'Angus and Alasdair.'

'How old?'

'Angus is six and Alasdair will be four in April.'

'Why the big secret?'

'Their mother left me when Alasdair was one and remarried before he was two. She doesn't let me see them much. I was such a mess at the time. I took the first job opportunity that came along and ran away to Kent. Little by little I've lost contact with them. It's me I'm ashamed of. I shouldn't have run away with my tail between my legs.'

'What's stopping you seeing them?'

'They call this other bloke "Daddy", there's not much room for me.'

'But you do want to see them?'

'Yes, yes, I do. I think about the boys every day but every day it gets harder to go back.'

'Do you want to go back?'

'Not to their mother, no. Please don't think that,' he begged me, grasping my hands in his.

'They're your children. Don't let someone else be their daddy if it's not what's best for them.'

'Isn't that selfish of me, stirring things up again?'

'I don't know, Danny. Is you being out of the picture better for your boys or is it easier for your ex-wife?'

'Why do you have to be so understanding?'

'I'm sorry?'

'I've already messed up my marriage and my relationship with my boys. What about us?'

'What about us? Don't use me as an excuse for not seeing your children.'

'I'm a coward really.'

'Most of us don't fight for what we want. Or even know what we want. We let life happen to us.'

'What do you want, Sarah?'

'Oh, I don't know,' I lied. But I did know. I knew every time I held a baby in clinic for just a second longer. I was starting to want my own baby, maybe not for a couple of years, but I couldn't deny that feeling. It didn't feel like it would be my turn anytime soon.

Trundling past The Old Goal, Mr Hopkins's residence, on my way back from Tuesday morning visits I spied Hermione calling with arms full of provisions for the invalid. I hoped their romance was developing better than mine; I'd seen neither hide nor hair of Danny since our Thursday night supper. It had been nearly a month since Mr Hopkins's near miss at the Burns Night ceilidh and without fail, come frost or sleet Hermione had been in to see him every single day. Apparently, Etty, Hermione's mother, was keeping the headmaster well stocked in stovies, Scotch pancakes and flapjacks to keep out the cold. The village was awash with gossip but barely a word passed Hermione's lips on the subject despite numerous attempts from Mrs Jefferies to wheedle information out of her when she arrived back at clinic for lunch.

'I suppose many men prefer to have a nurse as a wife to care for them in their autumn years. Much cheaper in the long run,' Mrs Jefferies attempted to bait Hermione.

'I dare say,' replied Hermione. 'Though there are nurses and nurses. I think a district nurse would be preferable to a health visitor, don't you?' she purred with her sweetest smile. At the reference to her husband's affair with the former district nurse, Mrs Jefferies stormed out of the office, nearly cracking the glass in the door as she slammed it. 'A saucer of cream for Miss Drummond,' Hermione tutted at herself.

'She's insufferable,' I complained.

'She was malicious. And that never pays,' corrected Hermione. 'Oh Lord, the fish van will be here soon and I've got a hearing test downstairs in five minutes.' She frowned, looking at her gold Swiss wristwatch.

'I'll go for you if you like?' I offered.

'Sarah, you're an angel. Would you get me two hen lobsters and four salmon steaks?'

'I'll drop them off at River Cottage on my way to Hollow Prospect.'

'A seraphim. You're definitely a seraphim,' praised Hermione.

'What does Etty think of Mr Hopkins?' I ventured. Now I was fishing.

'Nothing at all. I said to Etty when she moved in, "You have your life and I'll have mine and never the twain shall meet."' I gathered up my things. 'Did you say Hollow Prospect, Sarah, my dear?' I nodded. 'Is today the great escape?' she asked. I earnestly nodded again. '*Bene! Ben fatto! Buon lavoro!*' Hermione congratulated me. Then with a little whisper of explanation. 'Mr Hopkins and I are learning Italian together while he convalesces – it's *la bella lingua*.'

'Hermione, if I don't make it back in time would you cover clinic for me, please?'

'Of course, Sarah. Don't hurry back. It would be my pleasure. Let Miss Milstead enjoy her new home – it'll be one of life's lovely moments.'

Before going to Hollow Prospect I dropped off the fish as promised to Etty.

'Gosh, they let you wear short skirts in school these days,' remarked Hermione's aged mother at the miniskirt dress I was wearing with leather knee-high boots. I pulled at the hem of my coat to cover my knees, suddenly extremely self-conscious though I had on a pair of thick black tights. 'You girls are so lucky. I had such beautiful legs and I had to hide them,' Etty told me. 'Here's a few pennies. Get yourself a cup of cocoa. It's a chilly day and you might catch cold.'

I hovered in the lane to check the coast was clear at Hollow Prospect. I could see the small figure of Valerie looking out of an upstairs window of the rickety farmhouse. It was slippery underfoot as the uneven surface of the mud had an icing of frost on it. Before I got to the door Valerie flung it open. She'd already buttoned up her overcoat, and she thrust the baby tucked into a basket in my arms.

'Let's get going,' she told me excitedly, picking up two smallish grey suitcases. We walked gingerly to my Mini and put the bags in the boot. 'Two ticks, I've got a box with the baby's bits in,' she told me, trotting back to the house. Valerie reappeared a moment later with a cardboard box which contained a makeshift steriliser, a couple of bottles, milk and a few packets of flour. She steadied the box on her hip, slammed shut the kitchen door and marched back to me triumphantly. 'I had to secretly pack and hide everything under the bed,' she told me.

'Is that everything?'

'Yes, we haven't got much.'

'Are you ready?'

'Yes, I never want to set eyes on this miserable place again,' she told me. 'Let's get off quick before they come back.'

Off we sped out of the woods, over the hill and on to the road to Maidstone, far, far away from Valerie Milstead's horrible uncles. Chris Jentry was waiting for us with the keys on the doorstep of the 1950s council flat in the centre of town. Laid out on the lawn outside the two-storey little block was a white cot, a single bed, a couple of kitchen chairs, a table and a TV.

Valerie carried baby Michael to the door of her new home. 'What's all this?' she asked Chris.

'A mate dropped it off in his van for me but he had to get off,' explained Chris. 'I wanted you to be the first person through the door. Here, it's yours,' he told Valerie, handing over the keys to her flat. She stretched out a free hand and ran it slowly over every stick of furniture. 'It's second-hand but it's good stuff,' added Chris. 'Here, Miss Hill, let me give you a hand,' he called, jogging over and taking Valerie's box and another one I'd filled with blankets, sheets and pillows.

We all stood on the doorstep and waited.

'Shall I open it, Nurse?' asked Valerie.

'It's your home,' I encouraged with a smile.

Slowly Valerie put the key in the latch and gave her own front door a little push. We followed her in, Chris barely able to see over the boxes and me with her two suitcases. Valerie was silent as she gazed around at the empty sitting room. It had an old tiled fireplace and a gas fire. At least they'll be able to keep warm now, I thought.

'Shall I turn on the fire and get the place warmed up?' I suggested.

'Please, Nurse,' said Valerie, standing in the middle of the room and turning round slowly in a circle on the bare floorboards to take in her new surroundings.

I must see if I can find her a rug, I thought. The sitting room had a large picture window that overlooked the communal lawn, still strewn with our furniture. 'We don't have any curtains,' I frowned, looking at the afternoon winter sun streaming through the window. 'Mr Jentry, would you take the other end of the blanket and help me to hang it up at the windows for tonight?' I proposed, rooting around in the cardboard box for a blanket and some string to create a makeshift curtain. Once it was up we admired our handiwork for only a moment. 'Mr Jentry, shall we carry the furniture in and give Miss Milstead a few minutes to look around?' I suggested.

Once all the furniture was inside Chris plugged in the telly. 'It's only a black and white one, but you could always save up for a colour one,' he told Valerie.

'I haven't watched telly for over a year,' said Valerie. 'Can I watch *Rentaghost* later?'

'It's your TV, Valerie. You can watch whatever you like,' I explained.

'Can I really? How nice.'

We followed Valerie into the bare kitchen that opened up onto a little garden with a fence and a gate at the end.

'There's no stove or fridge, I'm afraid,' apologised Chris. 'But I'll try and get you a stove tomorrow. It might be a bit of a wait for a fridge.'

'Can I go outside?' asked Valerie, peeking out of the kitchen window over the sink.

'Yes, of course. It's your garden,' answered Chris.

'All for me?' she asked.

'All for you,' confirmed Chris with a smile. 'I'll be off now. But give me a ring if there's anything you need. I've left a note on the mantelpiece with useful numbers and a few coins for the payphone if you need it.'

'Thank you, Mr Jentry. Goodbye,' I said.

Valerie stared at him for a moment. 'How many bathrooms are there?'

'Just the one,' said Chris.

'How many bedrooms?' asked Valerie.

'Two.'

'One for me and one for Mikey?'

'You can keep Mikey in with you for now,' I advised. 'But he can have his own room when he's a bit bigger.'

'And no one else has a key or will be coming in?' pressed Valerie.

'No, Miss Milstead. This is for you and your baby. It's your home for as long as you want it.'

'And you won't tell anybody where I am?'

'Not if you don't want us to, Valerie,' I confirmed. 'You'll be safe here.'

'Thank you. I can't believe you did this for me. Do I need to give you anything, Mr Jentry?'

'Nothing at all,' said Chris. 'I've set up your social security, you'll get money every week for you and the baby. Your book will hopefully come in the post tomorrow. We might be able to get you something for some more bits and pieces.'

'Thank you. It's more than I deserve,' she cried.

'Everyone deserves to be safe, and warm and happy,' I told Valerie, gently putting my arm round her shoulder.

'Good luck, Miss Milstead,' said Chris lightly before shutting the door on us.

'I'll help you unpack but I'll have to be off soon, Valerie,' I explained, putting some food away in the cupboards. 'I'll pop in next week to see how you're getting on.'

'You can come anytime you like now, Nurse,' said Valerie cheerfully as she made baby Mikey up a bottle. 'But I'll stay clear of town on a market day, I think.'

'That would be a wise move. You can take your milk tokens to the Maidstone clinic now, it's not far. Take your medical card to register with the doctor's round the corner and I'll pass you over to the new health visitor.'

'But you'll come as well, won't you, Nurse?'

'I can't be your health visitor anymore but we'll keep in touch for as long as you'd like to.'

'You'll come and see me next week?'

'If you like.'

'Oh, I won't know what to do with myself with just this nice little place to keep clean. It's like a dream. Quick, Nurse, pinch me and see if I wake up,' she said with a giggle, offering me her arm. It was the first time I'd seen her laugh.

Four o'clock – teatime for the county set. I hoped Lady Cecilia Beauchamp-Smith would be enjoying a cup of Assam in the library but annoyingly I'd only had time to take my winter coat off and say hello to Mrs Reyes before her ladyship came bustling into the kitchen on the pretext of needing more hot water for the teapot.

'Here again, Nurse?' Lady Cecilia trilled while Cristina Reyes fetched and carried. 'Is there something wrong with the baby?

You're here so often you could almost be a nanny,' she half-laughed.

'This is my last visit. I'll see Mrs Reyes at the clinic once a month from now on,' I informed her.

'That seems a bit excessive,' said Lady Cecilia. 'I'm not sure I can spare you, Cristina. When is the clinic?'

'Thursday afternoon at The Meadows,' I said.

'But Cristina's afternoon off is on a Sunday,' responded Mrs Reyes's employer.

'It is in the best interests of the baby and her mother, Lady Cecilia. I'm sure you wouldn't want to risk their health?'

'Of course not. It is most inconvenient but if you think it necessary, Miss Hill, you know best, I suppose. But we can't spare José and I wouldn't want the Rolls going to The Meadows of all places.'

'There's a bus that will collect Mrs Reyes.'

'Oh, in that case I suppose I'll have to fend for myself for an hour or so. You make sure you hurry back, Cristina,' Lady Cecilia warned her housekeeper.

'Of course, Lady Cecilia,' replied Cristina, who'd been silent until now on the subject of herself and her baby.

'Tell the bus driver to drop Cristina off first. Thursdays are not her afternoon off. I'll take the teapot up myself,' Lady Cecilia announced magnanimously. 'We wouldn't want you tiring yourself out, would we?' She flounced out of the kitchen.

'Will the bus be expensive?' asked Mrs Reyes shyly.

'It's completely free. You won't have to pay a penny,' I assured her.

'That's good. It'll be nice to get away from the house for a few hours once a month. I never go anywhere.'

'When you get to clinic there'll be a free tea and biscuits too. I'll ask the driver to collect you from the end of the drive at 1.15 p.m.

and drop you at 4.45 p.m. You'll get three and a half hours to yourself.'

'It'll be like having an extra 12 afternoons off a year,' whispered Mrs Reyes.

'That's what I thought,' I colluded. 'The other mums are a nice bunch, very friendly.'

'I don't have any friends here,' lamented Mrs Reyes. 'If we were near family it would all be so different.' She looked utterly drained with the work of looking after such a big house and a new baby: it was too much. I didn't know how she did it. Crystal was a beautiful baby, growing well, with a gorgeous mop of thick black hair and active dark eyes that followed you everywhere. Mrs Reyes reached into the basket and held her daughter's chubby little hand. The kitchen door opened and she jumped away and started busying herself immediately picking up some mending from her work-basket but it was only her husband, fresh from the garden. His wife heaved a huge sigh of relief and put the mending back down.

José Reyes was a few years older than his wife. Tall, slim and quiet, he slipped in with barely a word and poured himself a glass of water.

'I've got to change into my chauffeur's uniform to take the Captain to Canterbury,' he grumbled.

Cristina reached in and picked up their baby for a cuddle, cooing over her softly, kissing her sweet soft head.

'Is the baby well?' asked Mr Reyes quietly.

'She's perfect,' I replied. Mr Reyes beamed with paternal pride and joined his wife to take a few moments to enjoy their baby daughter.

'We wanted a better life for our children, that's why we came here,' Mrs Reyes told me. 'But it's very lonely. I barely see José – the Captain and Lady Cecilia keep us so busy.'

'Life would be so different if we could only get to America,' added Mr Reyes wistfully.

'What's to stop you applying for a visa?' I suggested.

'Can we do that?' asked Mrs Reyes.

'I don't see why not,' I said.

'I don't think Lady Cecilia would like that.'

'It's none of her business – she doesn't own you,' I replied.

'But she could throw us out,' said Mr Reyes gravely. 'We'd be without a job and a home.'

'You don't have to tell her you're looking into it,' I tried again.

'She'd sniff it out,' said Mr Reyes.

'What if I sent for the forms and you filled them out at The Meadows baby clinic?' I proposed.

'Oh yes, José. Let's try. I want more for Crystal,' entreated Cristina Reyes.

'And then what?' asked Mr Reyes.

'You take the application forms to the American Embassy in London.'

'José, we have a little money saved. Let us try, please.'

'But how do we go to London? If we use the money for the visa then we don't have enough for the train fare to get to London and they won't give us time off to go even if we did.'

We all paused, frowning at the Reyeses' predicament.

'Do you ever drive Captain Beauchamp-Smith to London?' I asked.

'Sometimes,' said Mr Reyes with a shrug.

'Perhaps you could go to the embassy while you wait for him?' I suggested.

'Yes, José. At one of those regimental feasts he goes for,' pleaded his wife excitedly.

'There's not anything planned at the moment,' said Mr Reyes.

'But there will be one at some point?' I asked.

'Yes, I expect so,' he said.

'If I send for the forms we could fill in the application at the clinic to get the ball rolling?'

'Even if your plan works we can't afford to go to America,' he brooded. 'I need to get changed – dreaming doesn't pay the bills,' he muttered.

'But we can at least fill in the forms, can't we?' asked Mrs Reyes.

'We'll see,' conceded her husband as he went up the back stairs to their cold attic room to transform into the Beauchamp-Smiths' chauffeur.

'Don't you worry about him, Miss Hill,' whispered Mrs Reyes once her husband was out of earshot. 'I'll work on him. We're so excited for the clinic on Thursdays, aren't we, Crystal? It's going to be your first big adventure,' she murmured into her baby's ear.

As promised I called in to see how Valerie Milstead was getting on in her new flat. I took her some good-quality second-hand baby clothes, a few saucepans and her final home delivery of National Dried. When Valerie opened the door with Mikey on her hip they both looked better after only a week. Her fair hair was freshly washed and much lighter in colour than it had been at Hollow Prospect. I guessed her uncles had kept her short of privacy, hot water and toiletries. Valerie wore a striped multi-coloured jumper over blue flared jeans and Mikey had on a red and white striped romper suit. Both were pink-cheeked and bright-eyed without the runny noses and tickly coughs.

'I bought us some new things at Woollies,' Valerie said, beaming.

'You both look great,' I praised.

'I've seen more folk this week than in the whole time I was in Totley,' she told me, closing the door. I followed her through to the kitchen. 'It's so friendly here. Can I make you a cup of tea, Nurse?'

'That would be lovely, thank you.'

'It was so funny. There's an old lady across the hall, Mrs Groves. She knocked on the door last week to ask how we were settling in. I said to her, "Good. I'd invite you in for a cup of tea but I don't have any sugar." And before I knew it she'd dashed off and come back with sugar, tea and an old china tea service she said she didn't need any more and wasn't worth the dusting,' Valerie told me, pouring hot water into a floral teapot and setting out cups and saucers on the kitchen table. 'I feel like a proper lady, making you tea like this,' she said with a giggle. 'It does make us laugh, doesn't it, Mikey?' She grinned, tickling her baby's toes as she popped him into a highchair next to us.

'You've started weaning then?' I remarked.

'Oh yes. He's quite the greedy guts, aren't you, little man? I gave him baby rice like you said and he gobbled the lot.'

'Maybe you could try him on a few more teaspoons then?' I suggested. 'And add in some apple puree?'

'Oh yes. He loves his din-dins, don't you?'

'Two little meals a day would be just the job when you think he's ready. And before you know he'll be having three meals a day and little morning and afternoon snacks.'

'Righto,' she breezed. 'I feel like a different person. We've been getting such a good night's sleep. No coughing. No knocking at the door. No cold frosty bed sheets on a lumpy old mattress.'

'That's wonderful, Valerie.'

'And the people here are nice too. It's not all young mums, it's a real mixture. But there's another girl my age with a little boy. We went to Woollies together and the Wimpy. She persuaded me to get the clothes. We had burger and chips and a milkshake. It was so much fun,' she told me, slurping her tea. 'I've forgotten the biscuits,' she said with a titter, fetching a packet of custard creams from the cupboard. 'I think we'll be really happy here, Nurse. And when Mikey's a bit older there's a nursery just down the road. Maybe I could get a little job. As a waitress or even in a shop. Do you think I could work in a shop?'

'Yes, Valerie. I think you can do anything you like.'

She grinned at me. 'I knew you'd say that, Nurse. You see the best in people, don't you?'

Oh no, I don't, Valerie, but it's nice of you to say so, I thought.

When I left them for the last time it was like a weight had been lifted. To see them settled and happy, so different from when I'd first met Valerie and her baby in that autumn rainstorm. We both seemed to be finding our feet in our new lives in Kent and soon spring would be on the way.

# 20

Thursday, 14 February – Valentine's Day and no date. Danny had decided to go to Glasgow to see his boys, leaving me with no one to fill me in on *When the Boat Comes In* and enjoy a cosy supper with after my Girl Guide class. So, after weeks of requests from Laura to get our fortunes told by Queenie Dangerfield, we were en route to the gypsy camp at Mill Farm in Hermione's MG with an almost full moon high in the sky over Fairy Wood. We'd waited for Ernestine to join us but she'd been called out to a home birth for a third baby and was hopeful it wouldn't be too long and she'd make it back in time for a reading.

'Do you think she'll be able to tell me when I'll get married?' chirped Laura in the back seat of the MG.

'Surely, it's an "if", dear,' corrected Hermione.

Laura ignored her. 'People say gypsies can tell just by looking at you what your future will be. Do you think they make love charms?'

'Who would you use a love charm on?' I asked Laura, swivelling in my seat to get a better look at her.

'No one,' answered Laura a little too quickly, slouching down in the back seat. 'What about you, Hermione?'

'You know why they call it a private life, don't you, girls?'

'No, why?' answered Laura.

'Because it's private,' purred Hermione, turning down the track to Mill Farm. 'Did you bring illumination, Sarah?' she asked as we left the MG at the gate. I pulled out my trusty torch from my handbag and waved it. 'Excellent – let us follow the trail of breadcrumbs and see where they lead us.' We followed the path through the woods. Lisa-Rose was seated cross-legged at the campfire wrapped in a shawl on top of a huge blanket, listening to her father play the fiddle.

'Mammy's ready for you in the caravan but you'll have to go in one at a time or she'll get her wires crossed.'

'Can I go first?' Laura jumped in.

'I don't mind,' I replied.

'Youth before beauty,' Hermione assented.

Laura knocked on the door of the Dangerfields' Romany caravan. Queenie swung open the door, looking regal with a purple scarf woven around her head and a long red velvet gown with black elbow-length gloves. She wore a huge jet amulet around her neck.

'Enter Madame Arcati, stage right,' whispered Hermione in my ear.

'You're looking for a love charm,' Queenie told Laura, taking her hand and giving the palm a good pummel with her fingers and thumbs. 'You've got good flexible thumbs. I can see you've no chavvies yet but love is coming. After seven full moons have passed a man with a healing touch will have entered your life and you'll be needing a little bit of gypsy magic to help things along,' predicted Queenie. Laura was entranced, and entered to have her future revealed.

'Sit down and have a brew,' said Lisa-Rose, offering us each a mug in white and blue striped cups.

'What glorious china,' admired Hermione.

'Dad made them,' beamed Lisa-Rose.

'An artist and a fine musician,' complimented Hermione.

Moses Dangerfield's dark eyes twinkled and he pulled up a log next to Hermione. 'I can see you're a woman of both taste and beauty,' he flattered, taking up his fiddle once more to play a rhapsody.

'Missus, do you know the teacher in charge at the school?' asked Lisa-Rose.

'Mr Hopkins the headmaster, yes, I do.'

'No, that's not his name. Williams it was, wasn't it, Job?' asked Lisa-Rose, turning to her husband, who had joined us with the young lad who'd shouted at the ambulance.

'Weasely Williams,' butted in the lad.

'Mind your tongue, Billy-Boy,' scolded Job.

'What's this about that Williams fella?' asked Hermione. Her ears pricked up at the mention of Mr Hopkins's slightly irksome deputy.

'He's got it in for us gypsies,' said Job. 'He's got Billy-Boy and the other children on bread and water at dinner time.'

'He's what?' I was shocked.

'They didn't hand in their dinner money and rather than asking us he's put the children on nought but chaff and Adam's ale.'

'The dinner lady tried to give me a sausage today, but he made her take it out of my buttie and throw it in the bin,' added Billy-Boy.

'And it's not just that,' said Lisa-Rose. 'He's made all the children in the camp do games in their underwear.'

'Why?' gasped Hermione.

'He says they don't have the proper uniform for sports, but it's just to humiliate them.' That's too cruel – surely it was illegal, I thought.

'The children don't want to go to school and in truth we don't want to send them to be shamed,' explained Job and I could understand why.

'No, indeed,' sympathised Hermione. 'Would you like me to talk to Mr Hopkins? He's off sick at the moment but he'd never allow this.'

'We don't want to make things any worse. Perhaps it's a sign we should move on,' mused Lisa-Rose sadly.

'Hang on, don't rush into anything,' I suggested calmly but inside I was fuming; it wasn't right to let Mr Williams force them out with his barbaric behaviour. He should be arrested – wicked, wicked man.

'Perhaps we could arrange to give him a nice sharp shock,' proposed Hermione, arching a fine eyebrow in the direction of Ernestine, who was coming through the gate, still in her uniform.

'Sorry, I'm late,' called the midwife. 'Mrs Bourne went into labour at teatime,' she said softly to Hermione and me. 'But baby's all safe and sound.'

'Lovely – what did she have?' I asked, dropping my voice.

'A little boy. He's an absolute darling. She's called him Valentine,' she told us as the gypsy music sparked up again, masking our conversation.

'Gorgeous name,' approved Hermione.

Ernestine leaned in to whisper. 'We had a bit of a to-do, my sweetness. We couldn't get hold of Mr Bourne – he still doesn't know the baby's arrived.'

Oh, dear. I hoped Mrs Bourne was all right. She'd been at the back of my mind since the Burns Night ceilidh. We filled Ernestine in on the situation at St Agatha's Primary and Mr Williams's vindictive treatment of the gypsy children.

Ernestine shook her head. 'It comes to something when the teachers are bigger bullies than the kids,' she sighed.

'I did wonder if Bob would be best placed to pay Mr Williams a visit in his official capacity?' proposed Hermione.

'That would put the wind up him,' said Ernestine with a laugh. 'See how he likes having his collar felt by a bobby.'

'You read my mind,' chortled Hermione.

'I'll have a little word. Leave it with me,' Ernestine assured us.

Laura emerged from the charabanc with a rose bush in her arms, grinning like the Cheshire Cat. None of us asked her what it was for and she didn't say a word about her reading. It was my turn next. Queenie beckoned me with a crooked finger and I entered the caravan in trepidation. I didn't need the other side to tell me things were on the wane with Danny. Queenie lifted out a crystal ball from a hand-carved box and placed it theatrically on the table. Her hands wafted over the glass globe, then she closed her eyes and inhaled deeply through her nose and held her breath, her head swaying slightly before she opened her eyes with purpose to peer into the ball to see my future.

'I see two paths in front of you. One goes to sea and the other to land but there's also a third path. The way isn't clear yet – it's one you'll have to make for yourself. There's a lot of travel, people coming and going, but not you – you are like a tree that bends with the wind, gives shelter in the storm. Soon there'll come a time when you want to lay down roots. There's a man who's travelling away from you and I don't think you'll follow him. I see a child, a new child entering the world, the mother needs you, and an old friend who'll arrive without warning,' finished Queenie, putting the ball back in her box and getting out her well-worn large deck of cards to spread on the table. But I couldn't concentrate or remember much of what she said. Next time I'll bring a notebook with me and write it all down, I thought.

At the end as I crossed her palm with silver, she suddenly grabbed my hands excitedly and told me, 'I see a book with large letters on the cover. It's like your name but not your name. What's that?' How should I know, I thought. Queenie's predictions seemed like rambling guesswork to me. I was none the wiser.

At the end of the evening Ernestine gave Laura a lift and I went back with Hermione. 'How was your reading?' she enquired.

'Confusing,' I frowned. 'And you?'

'Apparently, I'm going to have a big event in a church,' chuckled Hermione.

'Like a wedding?' I ventured.

'There'll be a carriage pulled by horses with black feathers that will take me to the church.'

'Like a funeral cortège?'

'Perhaps it is Queenie's way of telling me I'm approaching an age when I'll spend more time at funerals than weddings,' said Hermione with a sigh. 'But let's not get gloomy. Divination is fun but it's not always an advantage to know what lies in store for us. We should live as much as possible – you never know when the fella in the sky will call.'

Hermione dropped me off. The garden of Ivy Cottage seemed otherworldly in the moonlight. I took a moment to admire all the vegetable beds I'd dug, the frosty hedgerows trimmed into place so you didn't get scratched as you passed by and the freshly painted potting shed Clem had helped me put up. It was becoming a little oasis of rural tranquillity. I couldn't wait for spring. Any day now the daffodils would be nodding to me as I walked up my garden path and shoots would start to appear from the earth – the garden was waiting to be woken up from its winter's dream. A fox ran by my garden gate and caused clucking in Clem's hen house next door but they were securely fenced. No fat hen for you tonight, Mr Fox, I thought. When I got back to the flat it was almost midnight and there was a note from Flo pushed under the door.

9pm Thursday 14 Feb
Dear Sarah
Woman with foreign-sounding name turned up with a baby
claiming to be your friend. She says she's come on a surprise
visit. She looks no better than she ought to be. Didn't want
to let her into your flat, said they could wait at mine.
Flo

Goodness, who could this be at this late hour, I wondered.
Perhaps one of the mums from The Meadows council estate? Flo
would recognise someone from Totley surely. I went with haste
to Primrose Cottage and knocked on the Farthings' door. On the
other side I could hear a commotion in the hallway.

'I can answer my own door, thank you very much,' chided
Flo.

'Calm down, pet. You'll give yourself a funny turn,' teased a
familiar Geordie voice.

Flo, with a face like thunder, flung open the door. Next to her
was a mature woman with bright blue eyes crinkled at the
corners. She'd grown out her wild curly hair and switched her
red lipstick to an orangey-pink gloss but that irrepressible smile
was unmistakable. It was Wade, or Edie Goldberg as she was
now, the tap-dancing midwife from my Hackney days. She'd
married Ernie the cabbie and had a late baby on my last day on
the wards.

'Edie, whatever are you doing here?' I hugged her, delighted to
see her again.

'So you do know her, then?' remarked Flo with surprise.

'She's my very dear, dear friend,' I replied.

'Told you,' added Edie, sticking out her tongue.

Mature as ever, I thought.

'Where's baby Jacob?'

'Asleep on Mr Farthing's lap on the sofa. Isn't he a lovely chap? So hard to find kind folks these days,' she said through gritted teeth, glaring at poor Flo.

'Get your things, Edie. Mr and Mrs Farthing need to get to their beds and so do I.'

Edie handed me a large red suitcase and ran back to collect her sleeping toddler. He slumbered peacefully with his head on her shoulder wrapped in a large blue blanket. Little Jacob must have been 18 months and had a mop of chestnut curls and pink round cheeks just like his mum. I took them to Ivy Cottage, hastily changed the sheets and put Jacob to sleep in my bed, so Edie could join him later. I'd have to spend what was left of the night on the sofa.

'What are you doing here, Edie?' I asked, putting the kettle on for a midnight cuppa.

'Aren't you please to see me, pet?'

'It's the middle of the night.'

'It was six o'clock when we left the East End.'

'Edie,' I pressed.

'We just needed a little break, that's all. And judging by those two next door your life could do with livening up a bit.'

'What does Ernie think about this?'

'He'll be glad to have a bit of time to himself, I expect. Or he will be when he gets off nights.'

'You didn't tell him you were coming?'

'I left him a note.'

'Oh, Edie.'

'He needs a shock. He takes liberties.' I didn't know what she meant and she didn't put me in the picture.

'How long are you staying?'

'Only a couple of nights, I expect. Anyway, pet, I'll skip the tea – it'll keep me awake and I'm that tired,' she informed me with a huge exaggerated yawn. 'I'll get straight to my bed. Night, night, don't let the bed bugs bite.'

She blew me a kiss and flounced off to my bedroom, to sleep in my bed without a word of explanation. Typical Edie.

# 21

Two weeks later and I still had my unexpected house guests with barely an explanation of why they'd come and when they were going. Sleeping on the sofa was giving me back ache. Hermione had offered me a bed at River Cottage but it seemed ridiculous to have to leave my own little flat and I didn't want to. It certainly wasn't big enough for the three of us and becoming a mother again had not improved Edie's housekeeping. She never picked up after herself, and soon my lovely neat home was awash with magazines, sweet wrappers, children's toys and cast-off stockings.

Danny had come back from Glasgow having seen his boys and we'd tried to have a meal together but Edie didn't do subtlety. She'd flirted outrageously, drunk most of the wine Danny had brought, turned up my record player to its loudest setting and grooved away to ABBA. I'm surprised the neighbours didn't complain. Danny had called me to ask if we could go for a drink at the weekend. I'd never been to his flat over the veterinary surgery in Malling and didn't think it would be a good time to start. I needed to keep my head clear and ask myself, as much as I liked him, was this what I wanted?

In the health visitors' office Laura and I were having a moan over tea and ginger biscuits. 'She must have said something about what happened with her and Ernie?' probed Laura, with her mouth full and dropping crumbs over my desk.

'Not a word. I don't know what's happened between them. He's rung a few times but she's refused to come to the phone. It's awful being in the middle of them. I don't want to answer my phone when it rings.'

'What about the little one?'

'Jacob's a sweet little baby but he's at that stage where he's pulling everything to bits. Edie doesn't take any precautions. I'm terrified he'll tumble down the stairs, or electrocute himself or set fire to the place while I'm at work. It's ridiculous – I'm a health visitor and I feel there's a child at risk in my home.'

'Sarah, I'm sure you're worrying too much,' said Laura, taking the last biscuit.

'Am I?' I shouted slightly. 'Yes, I expect I am, because I've not had a proper night's sleep for two weeks and my flat is a tip. This sort of thing was easier to swallow when I was a young nurse sharing digs, but this is my home she's invaded.'

'Oh dear,' sympathised Laura.

'I shouldn't be so ungenerous. Of course she's welcome and I want to help but I can't help if I don't know what's wrong, can I?'

'No, of course not. How does she seem in herself?'

'A bit quiet.'

'Is that unusual?'

'Extremely,' I huffed. 'When I leave, she's in bed. When I get home, I cook dinner but she barely touches it and takes herself off for an early night. At the weekend she stayed in bed and I took the baby out. He's a bit confused about it all, poor little chap.'

'Do you think she's ill or depressed?'

'I have been wondering if I should get her to go and see Dr Drake.'

'You know what it's like when you're a mum. You never get any time to yourself and she is on the older side. Didn't you say she's got a grown-up son?'

'Yes, he's in the navy. But Edie's a life force – she's got more spring in her step than most of us.'

'Maybe she just needs a night out. Why don't we take her out in Maidstone on Saturday night?' suggested Laura.

'I don't know. I was supposed to be going for a drink with Danny.' I thought back to the last time I'd been in a club with Edie and she'd disappeared to be discovered snogging a bouncer in the cloakroom of the Hammersmith Palais at a Tom Jones concert.

'See him on Sunday instead. I'm sure Flo would watch the baby,' continued Laura. 'I fancy a boogie. I had a rotten date last weekend. I need cheering up.'

'I thought we were trying to cheer Edie up.'

'Two birds, one stone.' She waved away my comment.

'Was it a man with healing hands?' I teased.

'No, it was one of the coppers Bob Higgins works with. I won't be seeing him again.'

'All hands?'

She nodded. 'Oh yes, and he was rude. I had on a new all-in-one bra slip. It did rather stop him in his tracks,' she said with a giggle. 'Frustrated, he left me on the doorstep of my flat saying every time I moved my underwear rustled like a packet of crisps.' We laughed. 'You never go out, Sarah – come on, let's ask her,' Laura enthused, grabbing my arm.

'What now?'

'No time like the present – come on,' she insisted, dragging me to Ivy Cottage.

'Edie,' I called as we went up the stairs. You never knew what you'd find when you came home. Yesterday, I'd discovered her attempting to clean the kitchen floor with two of my best tea towels on her feet, twisting away to Chubby Checker. 'You remember my friend Laura,' I trilled.

'We wanted to know if you fancied going dancing tomorrow night in Maidstone, if we can get a babysitter?' added Laura as we got to the top of the staircase.

Edie emerged from my bedroom still in a baby blue short nightie. 'A night on the town?' she asked. 'Do I ever!' she cried, stepping onto a kitchen chair in her stockinged feet and onto the kitchen table. 'Watch out, Maidstone, here I come,' she said with a laugh and then started to sing 'Hey Big Spender'.

Little Jacob toddled in. 'Mummy?' he said, looking up at me curiously. I nodded and picked him up for a cuddle. 'Mummy good?' he asked.

'It certainly looks that way, Jakey,' I replied with a grin.

I said goodbye to Laura who was off on her rounds. Etty Drummond had been suffering with a pulsating chest and tummy pains and taken to her bed. Hermione and Dr Drake had agreed she'd take more notice of the district nurse than her own daughter and to review her medication. Laura was popping in to take her blood pressure and talk to her about cutting back on the wee drams and fried foods, but she'd told me the 90-year-old was fading – we all knew the signs all too well.

Back at the office Hermione was on the phone with Ernestine at her elbow, bouncing up and down her toes in anticipation.

'Yes, we'll be right there, thank you, Mr Hopkins,' she finished, putting the phone back on the receiver. 'You're just in time, Sarah. We've got a few minutes to get a front-row seat at The Old Goal,' she said, mysteriously reaching for her coat and hat from the hat stand.

Ensconced in Mr Hopkins's bay window with a good view of St Agatha's we watched surreptitiously as a police car pulled into the primary school. Constable Bob Higgins got out, accompanied by a young policeman, and proceeded into the school. We waited for 10 minutes before the policemen reappeared, escorting Mr Williams, the deputy head.

'That's my cue,' said Mr Hopkins with a grin, before dashing out of his home and over the road to the school.

Mr Williams was shouting and little faces were popping up at the windows of the school to watch. The dinner ladies stood at the kitchen door with their arms folded, enjoying the show. As fate would have it, Job Drury came riding along on his father-in-law's palomino pony. Bob Higgins called him over and he joined them in the playground.

'I wish we could hear what they were saying,' said Ernestine.

I agreed with her, but we had better stay out of sight. Eventually, the policemen stepped aside from Mr Williams and Mr Hopkins shook Job Drury's hand, who then tipped his cap and rode off on his horse. The policemen got into their car and drove off, and I could have sworn Bob winked at us as he drove past the window. Mr Hopkins then proceeded into school followed by a forlorn-looking Mr Williams, while the dinner ladies had a good cackle and smoke before going back in.

'What do you think has happened?' I said.

'We'll have to wait to find out,' sighed Hermione. 'Back to work, ladies.'

We had to wait until five o'clock before Hermione's telephone trilled again with word from Mr Hopkins. It was just the two of us in the office. Hermione kept a straight face throughout the one-sided conversation, giving nothing away. At the end of the call she simply said, 'Thank you for letting me know,' and then continued with her notes.

I waited expectantly but she said not a word. 'Hermione, what was that?'

'A phone call, Sarah dear,' she teased. I glared a little. 'It was Mr Hopkins,' she revealed. 'He telephoned to let me know that Mr Williams is very relieved the gypsies won't be pressing charges against him.'

'Oh, how clever,' I replied.

'Indeed. Now he owes them. I'm expecting they'll all be having roast potatoes, gravy and veg followed by cake and custard for lunch next week. Because Job Drury saved Mr Williams's bacon and that will teach him.'

Yes, it would. Bob had told us it would have been hard to make the case stick if the gypsies had pressed charges but Mr Williams didn't know that. He thought without the generous intervention of Mr Hopkins and Job he would have been spending the night in a police cell and that was a lesson he would never forget, horrible little man.

Poor Edie. I don't think any of us had anticipated we'd end up in the ladies' loos with her in tears at 10 o'clock on the Saturday night. Huge rivers of mascara were running down her cheeks. She'd started off the evening with brandy and Babycham and all was well until a chap she was dancing with tried to kiss her. She'd slapped his face and run to the ladies' in floods of tears. Laura had gone to call a taxi – our night had clearly come to an abrupt end.

'What's the matter, Edie?' I asked.

'I'm just so ashamed of myself. When will I ever learn?' She sobbed, blowing her nose with toilet paper.

'Do you want to go home?' I asked.

'Yes, I do. Sarah, would you call Ernie and ask him to come and get me?'

'Of course. Let's go home and he can come and pick you both up tomorrow morning,' I reassured her.

'Do you think he will?' she whimpered.

'Edie, he's be calling you every day for two weeks and you've refused to speak to him. What's going on?'

'I'm pregnant again. At my age!'

'Aren't you happy about it?'

'Sarah, it's ridiculous. I thought it was the change this time, I really did. Flaming Christmas!'

'Edie, you're a midwife. You need to take more care.'

'I know, I know. But you know how it is. You're stuck at home for days, there's nothing worth watching on the telly, one thing leads to another and hey presto you're pregnant.'

'Do you want the baby?'

'Who knows – maybe I'll have a little girl this time,' she answered resolutely.

Ernie came to collect them at first light on Sunday morning. I was glad to wave them off but life certainly had more vim when Edie was around – she was a force of nature.

# 22

Mrs Mabel Dute, one of our clinic volunteers, let me into Kings Manor. I'd seen it from the road many a time but I'd never been over the threshold. It was a traditional house but with every comfort of modern life. The wall on the staircase was made of glass; as I followed the cleaner-cum-nanny upstairs I looked out onto an immaculate lawn, where little Antonia and Lizzie Bourne were playing in their sandpit.

'It's the first door on the right,' instructed Mrs Dute, pointing towards the balcony landing. 'I've got to keep an eye on the girls,' she called, running back to the hall and out to the garden through the conservatory.

I gently tapped on the bedroom door and Diane Bourne's demure voice beckoned me in. The mother-of-three was sitting up in a huge canopy bed, resting on large white fluffy pillows against a cream upholstered headboard. The shutters on the two sets of balcony windows were half closed. It was a beautiful airy room with buttercup wallpaper covered in green vines, a large wardrobe with glass doors and several large royal-blue velvet upholstered sunken armchairs. Mrs Bourne's rich auburn hair was held back with a white ribbon. She'd unfastened her lacy blush peach bed jacket and loosened her matching nightdress to feed baby Valentine.

Diane Bourne was such a glamorous woman, it looked like she had it all – beauty, money, a fabulous home, lovely children and a successful husband, and yet she stared blankly at her reflection in the dressing-table mirror while she fed without once looking at her new baby. There were no tiny touches or coos, and yet she did it, like she did everything, proficiently. Valentine was a bonny baby and feeding well, with a bright future ahead of him, just like his father.

The expensive perfume bottles and make-up were expertly arranged on Mrs Bourne's exquisite dressing table. The whole house was sumptuous and sparkling; it was like living in *Vogue* or *Vanity Fair* magazine and yet there was something missing. I couldn't put my finger on it, but something wasn't right.

'Do come in, Nurse. Pull up a seat,' she invited.

My leather boots made no sound on the thick deep blue and creamy yellow checked carpet. I moved the stool from the dressing table next to the curtained bed. They were both in the same fabric of cream with blue forget-me-nots. 'How's the last few days been, Mrs Bourne?' I asked.

'My husband was home. His family are delighted to have a boy. Poor Valentine – such great expectations and he's only two weeks old.'

'It can be very difficult coping with all the visitors when you have a new baby,' I empathised.

'You'd think Antonia and Lizzie were just the warm-up the way they're carrying on. I don't seem to be as excited as everyone else. He's no different from the girls; do we love them any less just because they have a brother now? I don't see why boys take precedence just because they have a penis. From my experience it's a hindrance; they follow that and forget both the head and the heart.'

'It's great you think of all your children equally.'

'I want him to grow up to be a good man, a good and caring and loyal husband. A kind brother, an affectionate son.'

'I'm sure he will be.'

She frowned a little. 'We couldn't get hold of Peter when I went into labour,' she recounted in a flat voice, detached from the information she conveyed. 'He said he had a book reading at the university, but when I called they said it wasn't until next month. I don't know where he was. He hasn't said.'

I didn't know what to say to her.

'But it's no use crying about it,' she continued. 'It won't help me or the children if I fall apart. I don't want any gossip. I don't want to be pitied.'

Mrs Bourne finished feeding Valentine and placed him in the hand-carved rocking cradle next to the bed.

'That's a beautiful crib,' I said admiringly.

'It's a Bourne family heirloom. Passed down from father to son. Peter's mother brought it at the weekend,' she told me without a smidgen of pride as she reached for her handbag on the bedside table. Diane Bourne produced a little bottle of pills. 'Dr Botten says I should take one when I feel sad,' she informed me, twisting off the cap and tipping a pill out into her palm. 'I can't remember the last time I felt joy. Not even when the midwife put Valentine into my arms. It was just relief. Not like when the girls were born, not at all,' she confessed, putting the pill onto her tongue and swallowing. She was like a bird who'd lost her mate, trapped within a gilded cage.

When I returned to the clinic Mrs King was at Hermione's desk with her diary open, making notes.

'Ah, Miss Hill, you come most carefully upon your hour,' she greeted me. 'Etty Drummond has been rushed into hospital and we must set to and cover Hermione's caseload.'

'Yes, of course. Poor Hermione. What happened?'

'A really bad chest infection. Doesn't look too hopeful. Your prayers would be appreciated at bedtime. But for now, let's see how best to split up this caseload,' suggested the spiritual and practical Mrs King. 'You had a rather mysterious phone call while you were out.'

'Really – who was that?'

Mrs King smiled indulgently. 'Wouldn't leave their name. Simply said, "Agreed, please send for forms."'

And she didn't ask me to elucidate on Mrs Reyes's message. At least there was hope their little family would be able to fly away from the big house.

On Thursday, Danny and I resumed our weekly suppers. We'd not seen each other much since his revelations about his boys, the trip to Glasgow and my extended house guests. Not wanting any more of his well-meant but bland fare I'd prepared a beam end pie of sliced potatoes, leeks and onions in a cheese sauce quickly after work and left it to cook slowly in the oven during my Girl Guide meeting. I fried us both an egg from Clem's hens in an attempt to increase our protein consumption with some early spring greens from my very own vegetable garden. Danny watched me admiringly while cuddling Ginger, who'd missed her tickles and strokes during our unintentional estrangement. Our pussycat did not appreciate the vegetarian diet and sloped off to see Flo next door for some chicken titbits.

'Och, you do spoil me, Sarah. Would you make me some of your stovies and tattie scones next week?'

'If you're still here?' I probed.

'Where else would I be?' he asked, taking from me a plate loaded up with a huge helping of pie. 'I'm not going anywhere. But I've been thinking about contacting a solicitor about seeing my boys a bit more often.'

'I think you should,' I encouraged.

'You do?'

'Absolutely.'

'You don't mind?'

'Not a bit. You need to see them regularly if they're to have a secure and loving relationship.'

'Thank you, Nurse Hill.'

'It's important, Danny. Otherwise children don't know if they're coming or going. Was their mum open to that?'

'No, she's not. Hence the solicitor.'

'That's a pity. Maybe she'll come round.'

'As far as she's concerned they've got a new daddy and she's got my monthly maintenance cheque. I'm just a walking wallet and an utter fool. Time to grow up and take my responsibilities seriously.'

I couldn't have agreed more. But there was now an undeniable ticking clock on our relationship.

# 23

It was gone two o'clock in the morning by the time I got to my bed and technically it was already Shrove Tuesday. Clem had called on me to assist him in the labour of Queen Bess, his beloved pig, the evening before. Danny had come over to watch Lesley Dunlop in *Our Mutual Friend* on BBC 2. Sometimes, I didn't know if it was me or my television licence that made him such a frequent caller at Ivy Cottage.

'Time to put your midwifery skills to good use, Sarah,' Danny had remarked.

'For your information, Veterinary, I am not nor have I ever been a midwife,' I replied airily. 'I am a health visitor.'

'No room for histrionics during farrowing, Nurse. Here comes the first little piglet – make yourself useful and dry it off,' he told me, handing me a small pink bundle of joy. Several hours later we had a litter of nine and Clem was ecstatic while Flo was already making plans for sausages, ham and bacon.

After a few hours of shut-eye I returned to Kings Manor to follow up on Mrs Bourne. Mrs Dute was tossing pancakes in a Le Creuset orange frying pan for the girls on top of a wide range in the sunbeam yellow kitchen with mustard cabinets and creamy wallpaper covered in red poppies. Antonia and Lizzie eagerly awaited their pancakes at the semi-circular wooden table attached to a long yellow counter that housed the kitchen sink. They twisted their tiny feet round the legs of the large button-backed leather ochre-coloured chairs. It was set with orange napkins folded into a neat triangle. Mrs Bourne sipped from a tawny owl coffee cup, watching the girls from the L-shaped wooden-panelled sitting room through an exposed brick archway that afforded a view of the kitchen. An arrangement of violets was in a silver vase.

'They're pretty,' I remarked, looking at the violets.

'Yes, a good-looking gypsy girl came to the door this morning selling them,' Diane Bourne told me.

'From the camp at Mill Farm?' I asked.

'Yes, though she said they'd be moving on soon. Peter thinks they're vagabonds but I've always thought they were quite romantic in their painted wagons. Free to go wherever they please,' she mused quite placidly.

'Where's baby Valentine?' I asked.

'Upstairs in the nursery.'

'Can we go and see him?'

'If you like,' she acquiesced and I followed up the staircase.

Valentine was awake and staring up at the high white ceiling of his nursery from his large wooden cot painted with scenes from Beatrix Potter. A slightly faded rainbow mural was painted on the pale-blue wall and silver ornaments lined the marble fireplace. I asked Mrs Bourne to undress the baby and got out my portable metal scales and blew up the inflatable cradle. Once we'd weighed the baby Mrs Bourne sank into a rocking chair and unbuttoned her blue blouse with white polka dots to feed. I went to the kitchen and returned with a glass of water for her and waited as she rocked back and forth until she was ready to speak.

'I've started ringing the Samaritans,' she told me. 'Every night when the children are in bed and Mrs Dute has gone home, and I'm all alone in this big house. I put on a cockney accent in case it's one of the worthy ladies so they don't recognise my voice.'

Everyone thinks Peter is such a golden boy, he was such a catch, but so was I. I used to be a fashion journalist, you know. I wrote for all the London magazines. I never thought I'd lose my husband to some floosy.' She paused for a while thinking over her life. 'I telephoned the university yesterday about the arrangements for this big christening Peter's family want,' she said. 'His secretary as good as told me he was out with that tart. When Peter eventually called me back I tried to keep calm but I ended up being hysterical. Crying and screaming. I could hear the disgust in his voice – he hates a scene. He told me not to expect him home this weekend – he didn't even bother to make up an excuse. And I've got no one to talk to. My parents think he's wonderful. If I told one of my friends it would be all round Kent by teatime and I can't leave him. What about my children? I don't want my marriage to be a failure – it's all I have. Does he think he'd have a better life than the one I've given him with some slip of a girl? What should I do, Nurse? Tell me, please?'

I thought for a moment and then suggested that though he might have had his head turned by this girl it probably wouldn't last. 'If you decide you want to keep him act the part of an independent woman who'll be fine without him, even if that's not how you feel on the inside,' I recommended.

'I could do that. I'll show him what he's missing,' she agreed, the colour coming back into her cheeks. 'I'm not going to sit around here waiting for him to leave me or not. His loss if he does,' she concluded, and I was glad she had.

As I walked back to the clinic down the Malling Road I could see the children doing pancake races in the field next to St Agatha's school. It was so good to see Mr Hopkins back at the helm, though he did need to take it a bit steady. I decided I could spare a few minutes to enjoy all the fun. Billy-Boy come bounding up to me, a medal round his neck. He told me with great pride he'd won his class race for the boys. I congratulated him and he pointed out Lisa-Rose and Job Drury watching from a corner of the field where a pony was grazing. Lisa-Rose had baby Fiance tied in a large shawl across her chest and was constantly kissing the top of her head and stroking her lovely thick dark hair. On Job's arm was a large empty egg basket.

'That's a fine basket,' I remarked.

'I wove it,' Lisa-Rose told me. 'Would you like one, Missus? I'll make sure I drop one round before we go.'

'Are you heading off soon?' I asked.

'Come April Fools' Day we'll be going down to the coast. The tourists will be coming back.'

'I'll miss you,' I told them fondly.

'Ah, not everyone thinks so kindly of us country people. We'll be back in the winter. Make sure you come and say hello.'

'I will, I promise.'

'Maybe you could do us a small favour?' proposed Job.

'If I can,' I replied.

'We've been keeping hens while we've been at Mill Farm,' he told me. 'We brought some eggs this morning to help with the pancake making. But we can't take all those birds with us. Would you take a few off our hands, Missus, for free, like?'

'I'd be happy to, thank you.'

'You'll be doing us a favour. I'll bring them round in the wagon in a couple of weeks. Would a Sunday afternoon suit you?'

'Yes, perfect.'

'We don't forget who's kind to us and ours. Good fortune to you, Missus. You're a real lady.'

I stood with the Drurys awhile and we watched as the older girls stood on the starting line, their faces smudged with flour from making the pancakes. Cecily Higgins, Ernestine and Bob's only child, was amongst them and she gave me a little smile. Ready, steady, go – Cecily was in the lead until she tripped over the foot of another girl. I wondered if it had been on purpose. My eyes flashed to her class teacher but she didn't seem bothered. Cecily picked herself up and finished the race, coming in last. The boys from class three were next. I saw the freckled face of Neil Bowyer. I must check on Jackie – she hadn't been to Mothers' Interest Group or Mums and Toddlers for a few weeks. I couldn't see her amongst the other stay-at-home mums from the village who'd come. I looked at my watch – maybe I could pop in on my way back to the clinic; it's only over the road after all, I thought. There was no answer when I rang the bell at the Bowyers' flat but I was sure I saw the net curtain twitch.

On Sunday Danny came over to help me build a coop for my imminent gypsy hens. He brought planks of wood and mesh in the Land Rover but before we'd finished unloading it the snow started to fall. Danny suggested we adjourned to The Good Intent to see what Ted had on the menu for Sunday lunch. We got a spot by the fire curled up at a round table enjoying roast beef and Yorkshire pudding. After dinner we were so cosy and comfortable we played shove ha'penny and settled down for the afternoon. I sipped port while Danny had lemonade as he was on call for the out-of-hours veterinary service. The snow kept on falling, covering Totley in a thick white blanket.

As the light started to dim Mr Hopkins entered the bar in his huge winter coat, shaking the snow from his hair. He looked anxiously about the saloon before spying Danny and me in the corner and came over to our snug table.

'I'm sorry for interrupting. I've already been to your cottage, Miss Hill, and hoped I'd find you here.'

'How can I help you, Mr Hopkins?'

'I wanted to make you aware that Miss Drummond got a telephone call that her mother was fading and has gone to the hospital. I wanted to go with her but she thought it would be best alone but I'm concerned about her, and I thought you ...,' he stumbled. 'I thought perhaps you ...,' he tried again.

'Of course I'll go. Danny, will you take me? Thank you, Mr Hopkins.'

We jumped to our feet, paid the bill and pulled on hats, coats, gloves and scarfs and hurried back to Ivy Cottage. We left the borders of Totley as the sun was setting, a ball of fire all the brighter against the shimmering whiteness of the Kent hills. Danny hung back in the waiting room while I went to find Hermione. A staff nurse showed me to Etty's side ward. Hermione sat at her mother's bedside holding her crinkly white hands in a snow-white hospital bed of crisp sheets. I touched Hermione gently on the shoulder.

'Ah, Sarah, I'm so very glad you're here. Etty slipped away about 20 minutes ago. The doctor has just certified her dead. I'll telephone the undertaker in the morning.'

'Is there anything I can do?' I asked, sinking into the chair next to my very good friend.

'I don't feel like driving – could you give me a lift home? I'll be ready in a few moments.'

I slipped away back to Danny and we waited until Hermione was ready to go. I offered to drive her back to the hospital in the morning to collect the MG. When we reached River Cottage I said goodnight to Danny and went in with Hermione. She poured us each a sherry in a fine little Edinburgh Crystal glass with a thistle etched onto it. We toasted Etty Drummond and sat together awhile by the fire. The snow had stopped falling.

'I do hope the frost won't mean the end of all the lovely spring flowers that have been popping up,' remarked Hermione.

'Daffodils might be lovely to have at the funeral and purple heather perhaps. Simple but beautiful, and hopeful.'

'That sounds perfect.'

'Since yesterday I've been praying to God to take her. I said to my father and aunts and uncles to please come and take her. I didn't want her to suffer. When the ward went quiet after visiting hours had finished her head went back into the pillows, and her eyes rolled up to heaven and all the light went out of her and I knew in that second she was gone, and I thanked the Lord for it. She was a wonderful woman but we knew it was her time to go.'

It was the end of an era for Hermione. The loss of a parent is always such a huge transition. As nurses, life and death was an everyday occurrence for us, but when it touches those you love, you grieve and pray and hope like everyone else. Hermione wanted to come into work but Mrs King and I insisted she have the week off.

We buried Etty Drummond on the Thursday; she had a funeral cortège of horses with black feathers on their heads just as Queenie Dangerfield had foretold.

# 24

'What are these 11 balls of marzipan on top all about?' asked Yvonne Underdown as we assembled to make the simnel cakes at the Mothers' Interest Group in the church hall in the run-up to Mothering Sunday.

'It's one for each apostle,' I explained.

'I thought there were 12 apostles?' queried Susan Bunyard.

'Yes, there were,' I began.

'But we leave off Judas,' interrupted Flo, a disproving note in her voice.

'Well, that's not very Christian,' muttered Susan. 'Still, he probably deserves it,' she concluded.

When we were packing away I asked Mrs Underdown if she'd seen Jackie Bowyer lately. She had not and I couldn't recall the last time I'd passed her in the street or seen her at the shops. I thought back to the previous afternoon in the church hall at Valentine Bourne's christening. I'd discovered Mrs Bourne hiding out in the ladies' toilets unable to face playing the happy wife any longer. She gripped the sink and stared at her perfectly made-up face in the mirror with disdain.

'Do you ever look at your reflection and scream without making a sound?' she asked me, opening her mouth into a wide O and screwing up her face in a noiseless cry. 'Sometimes I think, who is that woman staring back at me? I forgot to pick Antonia up from nursery Friday lunchtime. Isn't that awful? They telephoned and I had to pretend there'd been some domestic crisis but actually Mrs Dute had taken Lizzie and Valentine for a walk and I was watching the BBC2 test card of the little girl in the red dress playing noughts and crosses with that creepy clown. I should have been an actress – my whole life is one big performance. A perfect little doll in my perfect little house, taking little pills that make everything feel nice. But it's not nice. I don't want to be nice anymore. You're nice, Nurse. Where does it get us? Princess Margaret and Lord Snowdon are separating; marriage isn't till death us do part anymore. I threw my nice pills down the loo. Flushed them clean away. What will Peter say when I stop being so bloody nice?' she finished, taking her compact out from her handbag and powdering her nose.

'There's a woman who's started doing Swedish massage in the village. I've decided rather than screaming, crying or popping pills like sweeties I'll go to her once a week – see if that will loosen me up a little bit,' she added, before returning to the party.

Poor Mrs Bourne – it was torture waiting to see if her husband was going to leave her to live permanently in his mistress's love nest. I'd noticed how he played the doting husband so well in public at the christening, you'd never have guessed. They both acted their parts to perfection.

As I walked past Totley Garage I noticed the village-shop delivery driver taking a box to Mrs Bowyer. He knocked but she didn't answer. He shrugged and left the box on the front step. The shop was only round the corner, and then I remembered seeing the bread van from the bakery coming earlier in the week. Tomorrow I'll catch her as she's taking the kids to school and see what's going on, I thought.

\* \* \*

I watched from the window of Ivy Cottage with my mac on ready to leap into action when the Bowyer family emerged. It was after 9 o'clock and the school bell had rung – where were they?

Five minutes later the door opened and Neil and little Jenny emerged on their own, half dressed and eating toast as they ran down Main Street, already late for school. Jenny was only wearing a summer dress, and it was a drizzly day in late March. I know some parents sent their children to school on their own, but Neil and Jenny were still in Infants – I was sure Jackie had always walked with them in the mornings. Maybe she was finding getting four children and herself ready in the morning too much, I thought. It wasn't easy in cold weather with all the coats, hats and gloves to keep track of, but Jenny must have been freezing in only a blue and white checked cotton frock.

I dashed over the road. The Bowyers' door had been left ajar and I called up the stairs. There was no reply. I heard rustling and called again.

'Come up, Nurse,' Jackie Bowyer called down eventually. She was still in her dressing gown. Baby Gordon and Stacy were on the circular multi-coloured rug. 'I'm not feeling very well today, Nurse. I think I'm sick,' she told me.

'Oh dear, would you like me to make an appointment with Dr Drake?' I offered.

'No, I don't think I could make it to the surgery. I'm all hot and sweaty. Best I stay home until it passes.'

'When did you start feeling unwell?' I asked.

'It's been off and on for weeks now. Must be one of those bugs that lingers.'

'Have the children been ill?'

'No, they're right as rain,' she tried to reassure me.

'I haven't seen you at group or Mums and Toddlers for a while,' I commented.

'I haven't felt up to going out,' she told me, not meeting my gaze.

'When was the last time you went out, Jackie?'

'Oh, I can't remember now. Would you fetch me a glass of water please, Nurse.'

I went to the kitchen and ran the tap. Postcards from Trev's voyages were pinned to the cabinets. Jackie drank deeply. Her face was pale. I took her temperature but it was normal.

'Have you had any diarrhoea or vomiting?' I asked.

'You don't mince your words, do you, Nurse?' she said, attempting to cackle.

'May I take your pulse?' She snatched back her wrist. 'No, you can't. What do you want? Who asked you to come round with all your questions?'

'I'm sorry. Would you like me to leave?' I asked gently.

She paused for a long time, her breathing very rapid. 'I don't want to go to mums' things at the moment. I don't want to be the only mum who doesn't have a bloke,' she confessed.

'That's understandable,' I sympathised. 'Is it just that?'

She considered her answer. 'No, I don't want to go out at all. When I think about leaving the flat my heart starts going like the clappers – I can barely catch my breath,' she told me.

'Is that why the children have been going to school on their own and you've had all the shopping delivered?' I asked.

'Quite the lady detective, aren't you?' She tried to smile, a flicker of her facetious old self. 'Every morning I think I'll take them, but I can barely get out of bed. The kids have been having to get themselves ready. And it gets worse as the day goes on. I think, oh, I'll go out in a bit, and then I say to myself, oh, I'll leave it 20 minutes, and before I know it the kids have come home from school. When the little ones sleep I cry rather than doing something useful. Everything's blurry, I can't seem to get my act together. I can feel my heart thumping in my chest. It's going hammer and tongs, Nurse.' She pressed her hands to her chest. 'Is my heart going to pack in? Or am I going mad?'

'I really think we need you to see Dr Drake today,' I pressed.

'I can't go to the surgery, I just can't,' she buried her face in her hands.

'I'll get him to call here. You won't have to leave the flat if you don't want to,' I said softly.

She nodded in agreement. 'I hoped I'd just get better on my own. It's too much for me without Trev and I worry about him – every night I lie in bed worried he's drowned. I'm a terrible, terrible mother. They won't take the kids away, will they?'

'You're not on your own, Jackie,' I patted her arm. 'We're going to get you some help. This is not your fault – you're not a terrible mother; think of all you do for your children. They love you dearly and Trev will be home soon. How much longer till he's on leave?'

'Not for another four weeks.'

'That's not long. You're nearly there.'

'But then he'll go away again.'

'Yes, but then he'll be back for good. And in the meantime we'll get you some help. You're not on your own, Jackie.'

I went straight to Dr Drake and told him I suspected Jackie Bowyer had agoraphobia. After his visit that afternoon the good doctor concurred and did a referral to a psychiatrist to do a home visit at the end of the week. I popped in a couple of times. I listened to all the fears she'd been bottling up since the terrible night of the storm.

We waited together on Friday morning for the psychiatrist to come. Jackie kept popping to the loo every five minutes. 'I'm trembling all over, Nurse,' she told me, gripping the edge of the sofa. 'He'll take one look at me and put me in the looney bin. My throat feels all scratchy like it's closing up. Oh, I do feel faint.'

When the psychiatrist arrived I went to wait with Dr Drake at the doctor's surgery.

'What do you think he'll recommend, Doctor?' I asked.

'I expect he'll ask the mental health nurse to call with immediate effect.'

'They wouldn't send her away?' I let my own fears bubble up to the surface.

'No, no, no! She's not a risk to herself or her children as far as I could ascertain. The mental health nurse is a good woman. What Mrs Bowyer needs is regular support. Baby steps, Nurse. The mind is more of a mystery than the body. She needs time to heal.'

'I think she's worried people will gossip.'

'But going to clinic for treatment would be too much?' I nodded. 'We won't tell anyone. No one will know unless she tells them – they don't wear uniform. She could just be a friend.'

'But everyone knows everyone in Totley,' I frowned.

'If there's gossip the best thing is not to fuel it. They'll soon be onto something else. There's nothing salacious about the mental health nurse, I assure you. In fact, the watchful eye of our neighbours is more fixed to see if there are any visitations between River Cottage and The Old Goal, I believe.'

'Miss Drummond and Mr Hopkins?'

'I believe so.'

'What's there to gossip about?'

'What indeed?' fished the doctor, and I was glad I didn't know anything. Hermione had barely mentioned Mr Hopkins since Etty's funeral.

* * *

The warm glow of the morning sunlight felt heavenly as Danny and I worked in the garden of Ivy Cottage on Sunday. My boyfriend had come over to help me finish the hen coop just in time before Job and Lisa-Rose Drury drove down the back lane in a brand new pick-up truck with three black Marans and a beautiful wicker egg basket for me.

'That's a very nice truck,' said Danny, admiring the shiny red car.

'Do you like it? We got it on Friday. My father-in-law doesn't think much of it – he still prefers his wagon and nag, but I think it'll look just as sleek pulling our caravan,' said Job with a chuckle. We waved them off on their journey to the coast. Baby Fiance would be one by the next time I saw her.

'A life on the open road – do you fancy it?' said Danny wistfully.

'Don't you have to be getting off yourself?' I prompted. He had a long drive ahead of him to Glasgow for his monthly visit to see his boys.

'I don't think I'm going to be too popular being away this week. Lambing is in full flow,' he kicked a stone with his boot.

'I'm sure they'll manage without you.' I handed him a brown paper bag and a flask.

He peeked inside the bag and grinned. 'You made my piece and coffee – you're one in a million.' He kissed me, easily pleased with the jam sandwiches he liked so much. Danny got into the Land Rover and started to pull on jumper after jumper and wound all the windows down.

'It's such a warm day, what do you need all those woollies for?' I asked.

'It's a long drive. I need the windows open to keep me awake. You wouldn't want me to catch a chill, would you?' he said with a smile, pushing his auburn hair out of his eyes.

'You need a haircut,' I told him.

'Will you give me a wee trim when I get back?' he asked.

I nodded and kissed him through the window of the Land Rover. He switched on the engine and I could hear him singing 'The Bonnie Banks o' Loch Lomond' as he drove away down Main Street. I inhaled the sweet smell of freshly cut grass from the fields behind the row of cottages, glad that spring had finally come to Totley.

The visa application forms were all ready for Mrs Reyes when she came to the April baby clinic at The Meadows. I'd phoned the American Embassy and had them sent to me. Together we started to fill them in at my consultation table in the corner. I desperately wanted them to get away from the Beauchamp-Smiths.

'The Captain has a regimental lunch in London at the Dorchester on 1 June,' Mrs Reyes informed me.

'That's very near the American Embassy. Shall we try and arrange an interview for then?'

Mrs Reyes nodded. 'I feel like Lady Cecilia is watching me like a hawk. If she finds out, she will sack us,' she whispered.

'I'll see if I can make the appointment. You'll have to watch out for the letter from the embassy. Who collects the post?'

'I do. But I'm not allowed to use the telephone. Would the embassy tell them we've applied?'

'I don't think so. You'll have two months to prepare for the interview. Will you be able to get everything in order by then?'

'Do I have to go to the embassy too?' she asked.

'They'll want to interview you both.'

'Oh dear – she'll never let me go.'

'Don't worry, I'll think of some excuse. Let's wait and see if we can get an interview on 1 June. Do you think it'll be easy for Mr Reyes to slip away?'

'Yes. They last for hours. José has to sit in the car and wait for hours and hours.'

Typical, I thought. He's there lapping it up at a posh hotel and his driver is left in the car all day because he won't put a few pennies on the meter.

'Do you really think we can do this? Get away to America?' Cristina asked me, her eyes large at the prospect of a new life.

'Yes, I do. Use this time to get everything ready. Mr Reyes needs to complete his section of the forms. You'll need to take your passports, photos and money for the visa. Do you have all that?'

'Yes, I can get those ready.'

'Good. You'll also need to show you've got enough money in your bank account to cover your expenses while you're in the States. Take your bank statements with you.'

'I think we have just enough. I will save every penny.'

'Your sister will need to send a letter saying she's happy for you to use her home as your residence.'

'I will write to her this evening. That will not be a problem. She really wants us to come.'

'Excellent. Fingers crossed for the 1 June, Mrs Reyes.' I filled in her notes, like it was just any other chat at baby clinic, and smiled. 'I'll see you at the May clinic but get word to me if you need anything in the meantime,' I whispered. 'Please do stay and have tea and biscuits. The bus will come to collect you at four o'clock,' I finished, as the next mother came forward and took a seat for a chat.

They have to get away, they just have to, I hoped.

# 25

The good people of Totley had gathered on the village green for the first cricket match of the season. Mr Bourne had returned to open for our village team against Malling and even Danny looked smart in his whites rather than his usual wellies and jumper. Once we'd helped serve the teas Lady Cecilia insisted all the ladies adjourn to the pavilion to discuss the summer fete.

'Isn't it a little premature to be making arrangements now?' said Mrs King. 'The fete isn't until the end of August.'

'And it does not organise itself,' snipped Lady Cecilia. 'Shall I put you down to judge the beautiful baby competition, in your professional capacity, Mrs King?'

'I usually do the scones,' replied my sensible colleague with a smile. There was no way any of us wanted to pick out who had the most beautiful baby – it was professional suicide. Judging the jam making at a recent WI meeting had been uncomfortable enough for me. I could have sworn several of the leading ladies of Totley had looked daggers at me for weeks afterwards.

'Miss Drummond?' enquired Lady Cecilia.

'Yes,' asked Hermione, who'd purposefully not been paying attention.

'Beautiful baby?' said Lady Cecilia, her exasperation mounting.

'I was rather bonny, yes,' teased Hermione.

'Would you be a judge?' snapped Lady Cecilia.

'No, no, no. Sweet peas on a soup plate is more my cup of tea,' responded Hermione. 'Put me down for that.'

'Very well,' said Lady Cecilia, noting it down on her clipboard. 'Miss Hill, that leaves you.' I looked pleadingly at Hermione and Mrs King.

'Mrs Jefferies as a senior colleague would be more suited to the task,' suggested Mrs King. Thank you, oh, thank you. Anything but the beautiful baby, I thought. We'd have to butter up Mrs Jefferies next week.

'Indeed,' barked Lady Cecilia. 'That leaves you with the WI best jam in show instead, Miss Hill.'

You can't have everything, I pondered.

One by one the ladies drifted out of the pavilion except Mrs Bourne. She looked very glamorous in a green and white striped wrap dress teamed with a large cream floppy hat. While Mr Bourne was batting I'd noticed the Honourable Bertie Beauchamp-Smith, Lady Cecilia's son, sidling up to Diane Bourne. She looked wonderful and he wasn't the only man who'd noticed her. Mr Bourne took his eye off the ball, then threw down his bat in a fit of pique and stormed off the pitch when he was caught out.

'How's your week been?' I asked Mrs Bourne as she sipped tea elegantly from a pink china cup balanced on a delicate saucer.

'I've changed the locks,' she told me, biting her bottom lip in a supressed grin. 'After Valentine's christening I said to Peter, if you feel you'd be happier with her then go. I'll do the best I can without you. When the locksmith came I told him I'd lost my keys, I didn't want any gossip. We've not told Peter's parents yet. When he came from his love nest in town this morning he had to ring the bell,' she said with a laugh. 'We were in the middle of a full cooked English breakfast before church. Peter fell onto the sausage and bacon ravenously, helped himself to coffee and told me he's not had a home-cooked meal for a month. He actually expected me to sympathise with him. Apparently, though, it's all very exciting – but she doesn't wash or iron his shirts, there's never any food in the cupboards, when he tries to make himself a cup of tea the milk is off and if he wants a bath he has to scrub the tub first.'

Eyes wide at this revelation I asked her, 'What did you say?'

'I didn't say poor you, have the benefits of being with that slovenly slut worn off so quickly? No, I didn't say that,' she said with a smirk. 'I said, maybe she's too busy,' and left it at that. You'll notice his cricket gear today is under par – not whiter than white as usual.' Mrs Bourne finished her tea. 'He's angling to stay the night, but I shall disappear and take the children out for the afternoon. He'll have to go back to his paramour in London and lump it,' she said with relish.

Bravo, Mrs Bourne, I thought. How's that?

On the village green, Mr Hopkins was bowling. I cast my eyes over to Hermione, who was sitting with Mrs King in deckchairs, children lying at their feet. Under a tree, Jackie Bowyer sat on a rug with a picnic laid out. Trev was home on leave – he played with Stacy while Jackie plaited Jenny's hair. Neil was pushing baby Gordon around the field in his pram, trying to get the baby off to sleep. Jackie Bowyer saw me and gave a little smile, but I didn't want to interrupt their time together. It was amazing to see her out at all. The mental health nurse had been working with her to come down to the street at first and last week I'd seen them walking together to collect the children from school. Trev's return had given Jackie a boost – he said he'd known something wasn't right by her letters. The Bowyers would have four weeks together before Trev would have to go back to sea for one last voyage. I prayed it wouldn't be so hard on Jackie this time, but perhaps it was best to enjoy the sunshine and worry about that when the time came.

Mr Hopkins made a run, spinning the ball rather well. He stopped suddenly and grasped his side. Hermione was on her feet in a flash, running over to him. I could see all the colour drain from her face; we all held her breath. I ran over to see if I could help.

'Dylan, are you all right?' Hermione asked.

'It's all right, it's only a stitch, and a complete and utter embarrassment,' replied Mr Hopkins, patting Hermione's hand.

'Thank heavens for that,' gasped Hermione.

'Do you think you could help me to one of those deckchairs, Hermione, my love? I'd prefer to sit out the rest of the match with you, if I may.'

'Of course you may.' Hermione beamed, taking his hand. Together they walked back to the deckchairs with every eye in Totley on them, and they didn't care a bit.

Bob Higgins took up Mr Hopkins's place and bowled out Malling's star player. Ernestine cheered wildly, and we all settled down for a blissful afternoon in the English countryside.

Mr Hopkins had called Hermione 'my love'. How very nice that sounded, I reflected. Did Danny love me, I contemplated, as I watched him field. If he did decide to go back to Glasgow, would I be heartbroken? I liked him very much, but if you loved someone, didn't you know it?

# 26

Walking hand in hand, Jackie and Trev went into the village hall to vote. Election days were funny things – everything could change and yet life carried on as normal; Clem in his keeper's suit tending to the bees, me on the way to baby clinic at The Meadows in my green Mini, filled with hope that Mrs Reyes would have an appointment at the American Embassy.

'It only came on Monday,' Mrs Reyes said, beaming as she passed me the letter. 'We have our interview on 1 June at one o'clock.'

'What time does Captain Beauchamp-Smith's function start?' I asked, reading through the instructions carefully.

'Twelve o'clock.'

'That's perfect. You need to be at the American Embassy with all your documentation at 12.30 p.m. You should be finished by 4 o'clock at the latest. What time does he usually finish?'

'Oh, he'll be drinking in the hotel bar till after 5 o'clock. Then he usually goes to his club on Pall Mall for dinner and José drives him home about 10 o'clock. They usually get to Totley Grange at midnight so poor José has to pay for his food if he wants something and London is very expensive – sometimes he doesn't have a thing.'

What a long day for poor Mr Reyes, I thought and how typical of the Beauchamp-Smiths that they were such slave drivers. 'Why don't you pack a picnic for you both and sneak it into the boot of the car,' I suggested. 'I'll pick you up a little after nine o'clock in the morning and drop you at Totley Station – that should give you plenty of time to get to London for the interview. Do you know how to take a bus from Charing Cross to Park Lane?'

'José will pick me up from the station once he's dropped the Captain and then take me back again.'

'Perfect.'

'Will you be able to collect me from the station? I don't know exactly what time the train will get in.'

'Don't worry, I'll wait for you from 5.30 p.m.,' I reassured her.

'You're very kind, Miss Hill. I do hope nothing will go wrong.'

'I'm sure it won't. Do you want me to write it all out for you?' I asked, picking up my notepad and pen.

'Please, there's such a lot to remember.' I started to scribble down a timetable and checklist. 'What do I tell Lady Cecilia though? She won't be happy about me having a day off.' Mrs Reyes grew anxious again.

'I thought you could say you need to take Crystal to Maidstone Hospital for some checks and that I've offered to take you there and back again.'

'She won't like it.'

'Probably not, but I don't think she'll object if she thinks it's official,' I guessed and I was right. Everything was in place. We just needed the embassy to give them a visa and then we could plot their escape from Totley Grange.

Only a week had passed since Trev Bowyer had left for sea and I noticed the bread van had started calling again. I telephoned the mental health nurse – she hadn't been in for a month. Jackie had been adamant she was better and didn't need any more help but after a call from Mr Hopkins to alert me that Neil and Jenny were coming to school on their own again we guessed the agoraphobia had come back. When I called at the garage, Jackie was reluctant to let me in.

'I don't want everyone thinking I'm loopy.'

'Do you not get on with the nurse?' I asked.

'No, she's right enough. It's all the little nudges and winks you get when you pass people in the street. You know they're thinking there goes poor Jackie, she's losing her marbles, or worse. Look, I know you're trying to help, Nurse, but the kids will be home from school soon, and I don't want this raking up again. When Trev gets home it'll all go back to normal, I know it will.'

'That's not for eight weeks,' I protested.

'Six weeks or so,' Jackie corrected me. 'And it's half-term next week. So, really it's only five.'

I didn't know what to do. As I left the flat I noticed Neil picking a dandelion clock from the kerb on the corner of Totley Hill outside the village shop just as Bertie Beauchamp-Smith's car came tearing round the corner. He clipped the boy, and knocked him off his feet. I ran to help Neil. The little lad was shocked and crying but nothing seemed to be broken although he'd had a nasty bump to the head that would have to be checked out straight away. Quickly a crowd gathered round us and Bertie got out of the car claiming the child had emerged from nowhere and trying to slope off. I asked Mrs Seaton to go to the clinic and get them to phone an ambulance and the police, and to knock at the Bowyers' door to fetch Jackie. Poor Jenny was crying on the pavement next to us as well, both children crying for their mummy. Soon it felt like everyone in Totley was out on the street except Jackie Bowyer.

Mrs Seaton whispered into my ear. 'She won't come, said she can't leave the little ones. I said I'd have them but she refused and shut the door on me.'

The ambulance arrived and still Jackie hadn't come to go with Neil to the hospital. Mrs King sat with him in the ambulance and tried to soothe Jenny while I went to try and rouse Jackie.

'I'm sorry, Nurse,' Jackie wailed. 'I can't go out on the street. I saw from the window everyone standing there. They'll all think it's my fault, I'm too ashamed. I feel sick, I won't make it out the front door, it's all too much.' She returned to the window to look at the crowds. 'The police are there now too. They'll think I'm an unfit mother. All the kids will be in care by teatime if I leave the flat. I can't get to Jenny and Neil but if I stay inside I can keep my babies with me.'

She really wasn't thinking straight at all. If I could get the ambulance onto the garage driveway perhaps we could get her from the door into the vehicle in only a few steps. I suggested the plan. She didn't answer.

'They're crying for you, Jackie,' I said softly.

'Would you come with me, Nurse?'

'Yes, of course. Shall I ask Mrs Seaton if she can have the girls and we'll bring Gordon with us?'

She nodded.

'Only if the ambulance backs right up,' she agreed.

'I'll make sure it does. I'll just be a few minutes. Get yourself sorted. I'll take Stacy with me,' I said, gathering up the toddler in my arms. 'Jackie, I think I'd better see if I can get the mental health nurse to meet us there, don't you?'

'Yes, Nurse. I do need some help,' she murmured as she went into the bedroom to get dressed and then she shouted, 'And so will that Hooray-Henry when I get my hands on him!' She turned in the doorway. 'I'll bet you've never seen someone go funny like this before, have you?' she said sadly, the anger fading away as quickly as it came.

I hadn't, but there would be many more women like Jackie –

she wasn't crazy or a bad mother, she just needed help to get her feeling well again. Dr Drake was so right: the mind and our feelings are much more complicated than healing broken bones.

The mental health nurse met us at the hospital. Jackie threw her arms around her neck and wept. 'I thought you'd think I was a complete failure if I told you it had come back,' she cried, but agoraphobia couldn't just get better like that – it was understandable that during times of emotional stress it would be there. Miraculously Neil was fine, with no broken bones and only a minor concussion. I'd followed the ambulance on in my Mini and late that night I drove Jackie and her boys home.

'The girls will be asleep now too,' she told me, tucking Neil into bed. Gordon was slumbering in my arms. 'I'll phone Lynda Seaton early tomorrow morning and ask her to take Jenny to school. Neil can have a day at home. Then I've agreed with the nurse that I'll try and take them to school every day, even if I only manage a few steps. We'll get there. I could have lost my boy today and I couldn't even go to him, I was so afraid. It's like fear has become my fear. That doesn't make sense, does it?'

She laughed at herself, but it made perfect sense to me.

Over the bank holiday weekend there were ructions at Kings Manor. Mr Bourne, fed up with his lack of creature comforts, had tried to return home, thinking Mrs Bourne would welcome the wandering philandering husband with open arms. Instead his wife had refused to admit him. We went up to the nursery so Mrs Dute and the girls couldn't hear us.

'It felt marvellous. He grovelled on the doorstep, got down on his knees and begged me to take him back,' Diane Bourne told me, flicking her bouncy auburn locks. 'I told him to pick himself up, not to be so pathetic and not to make a scene in front of the children. I told him to go back to London and check himself into a hotel, then I might come and see him on Monday for lunch if I could spare the time.'

'And did you?'

'Oh yes, I breezed in after going to the hairdressers on South Molton Street. I felt wonderful. Peter, on the other hand, looked crestfallen and I must admit I didn't like seeing him like that – stupid fool that he is, I do love him. He told me he'd been having a midlife crisis and as soon as he moved in with her, he realised it was a huge mistake, that she was a silly, slovenly girl and that he'd been a complete idiot. I told him he'd made a mockery of all I do, taken me for granted and not treated me with any respect. Then he cried, right in the middle of Simpson's.'

I didn't feel any sympathy for him but I could see Mrs Bourne would take him back and she knew better than me what was best for her.

'I'll make him wait until Wimbledon starts. The university always gets great seats and I do like Jimmy Connors's legs,' she said with a giggle. 'I can almost taste the strawberries and champagne now. It's been a rotten 1976 so far, but summer is almost upon us, Miss Hill, and I'm feeling surprisingly optimistic.'

The bus had delivered all the mums and babies to The Meadows baby clinic but Mrs Reyes wasn't on the bus. I'd taken her to and from the station as planned on Tuesday and it all seemed to go without a hitch. Lady Cecilia was a bit sniffy about how long we'd taken when I dropped her back at Totley Grange but I don't see how she could have known about Cristina Reyes's trip to London unless someone had spotted her on the train or at the embassy. But did county ladies gossip or even notice other ladies' servants? I hoped not.

After clinic I had to know the Reyeses were all right, that our plans hadn't been discovered and they'd not been turned out into the street. What if they'd lost their jobs and didn't get the visa to America? What if I'd pressed them into making a horrible, horrible mistake?

Filled with trepidation I drew up outside the large forbidding gates of the Beauchamp-Smiths' home. I saw Mr Reyes mowing the lawn and waited until he noticed me. At least they were still here – they hadn't been sacked. José Reyes looked over his shoulder and then nervously came to the gates.

'Come round to the tradesman's entrance and I'll meet you there with Cristina,' he instructed me.

I drove my Mini down the track, bouncing in and out of potholes, and waited for them to emerge. 'Is everything all right?' I asked.

'Lady Cecilia is in a terrible mood,' Mrs Reyes told me. She looked rather wan. 'The mother of the boy Master Bertie knocked down is pressing charges for dangerous driving. Lady Cecilia's taken money out of my wages for Tuesday and says I can't come to the baby clinic anymore. We aren't allowed the use of the car on Sunday afternoons unless we pay for the petrol and we can't afford it. I'm too tired to walk five miles and back to the village – I can't do it,' she told me despairingly.

'I'm sorry. But she doesn't know about the embassy visit, does she?' Mrs Reyes shook her head. 'That's something,' I comforted. 'Do you need anything?'

'No, but it will be very difficult to meet you and I can't use the telephone. How will I let you know if we get a visa?'

'I'll drive by this gate once a week at this time. Do you think you could slip out and update me?'

'We will,' agreed Mr Reyes. 'Poor Cristina can't even leave the house anymore. It's become her prison.'

'I've been thinking, they took our fingerprints at the embassy – is that bad?' asked Mrs Reyes.

'No, no, no! It's just standard procedure to check you've never been in trouble with the law.' The Reyeses exchanged a worried look. 'You haven't have you?' I anxiously enquired. Should I have asked this question before now?

'There was a house guest last year. A great-aunt of Lady Cecilia. She said I'd taken an antique brooch she'd borrowed off her ladyship. But I didn't. She threatened to report me – I think it was a bluff but Lady Cecilia called the police,' confessed Cristina.

'But you weren't charged?'

'No. Mr Higgins came to investigate. A week later he discovered it in a pawn shop in Canterbury. The shop owner said a posh white lady had brought it in, so they had to let it drop.'

'I don't think that's anything to worry about,' I reassured her. 'Fingers crossed a letter arrives giving you a visa very soon,' I added, getting back into my car. 'Don't forget, same time next week,' I reminded them, before driving again very slowly down the track, hoping I wouldn't come across the Captain on Dash.

# 27

Summer was so hot that every time I got into my Mini I could barely sit down or put my hands on the steering wheel. I tried covering the wheel with a rug but it only minimally served to alleviate the heat. As I went on my rounds the butterflies fluttered in the swaying wheat and barley fields, dragonflies hovered over the ponds laying eggs, newts basked on rocks in the sunshine, and Danny and I feasted on strawberries and asparagus until we tired of such delicacies during the long light evenings in the back garden. Ivy Cottage was baking at night – I had to sleep with all the windows open.

June turned to July, the summer holidays were almost upon us and apart from a round of nits followed by chicken pox at St Agatha's Primary, the sun smiled on Totley. It was sports day on the last day of term and Hermione and I had been asked to hand out the prizes, which to me seemed like pure favouritism on Mr Hopkins's part.

The previous afternoon my weekly vigil at the tradesman's entrance of Totley Grange had been rewarded. A letter had arrived from the American Embassy granting Mr and Mrs Reyes a six-month visa. Mrs Reyes had immediately written to her sister to ask her to book an airline ticket. I brought Hermione into my confidence – I felt we'd need an ally in plotting their escape.

'What are they short of?' the ever-practical Hermione asked me once we were alone in the office.

'The rail fare, suitcases and clothes. They only have their faded uniforms and a change of clothes for Sunday.'

'I think you and I can run to that,' Hermione generously offered.

'Thank you, that's very kind.'

'Helping others is one of life's greatest rewards,' she remarked.

'Do you have a plan for spiriting them away? Are the Beauchamp-Smiths sojourning in the south of France only to return to find the house shut up and the servants gone without so much as a by-your-leave?'

'No such luck. They're here for the whole summer. I had thought they would be very distracted on the day of the summer fete,' I suggested. 'That would give Mr and Mrs Reyes the chance to save up a few more weeks' wages and get everything in order.'

'Sarah, that's brilliant. Operation Runaway is go. Shall we make our way to the school? It's almost one o'clock – they'll be starting soon.'

We sauntered out of the clinic, excited with our plans. Totley Garage looked marvellous, decked out with balloons and a banner that said 'Now Open'. Trev had returned from the sea permanently and reopened. Jackie was getting a little better week by week, and most days she made it to the school and to the shops. She said she'd try and come to Mums and Toddlers again the next week. We all missed her.

Trev was washing a car on the forecourt. Hermione couldn't resist going over to see him.

'I hope you're using a bucket and sponge and not a hosepipe to keep your vehicles shipshape, Seaman Bowyer,' she enquired. 'There's a hosepipe ban, you know.'

Trev pointed to his T-shirt with a cheeky grin. 'I'm doing my bit,' he said. His T-shirt had the slogan printed in large letters:

'Save Water: Share a Bath with a Friend'. 'I didn't like to ask but if you're offering, Miss Drummond.'

Hermione laughed. 'You can give my MG a bit of TLC.' She threw him the keys.

'It'll be ready by three o'clock for my most enchanting customer.'

Sports Day was lots of fun. I especially enjoyed the infants' races that involved dressing up, obstacle courses and building towers of bricks. When the last child had left brimming with excitement at the long summer holiday stretching out in front of them, we returned with Mr Hopkins to his office.

'I'm very much looking forward to the holidays for the first time in years,' said the headmaster.

'I thought you would have been counting down the days. Have you made any plans?' I asked.

'Not yet,' smiled Mr Hopkins, looking purposefully at Hermione.

My friend, usually so at ease, fidgeted uncomfortably in her seat and pretended to look at her watch. 'Goodness me, I must go and pick up my car from Totley Garage. It's nearly five o'clock – they will be closing soon. Enjoy your holidays, Mr Hopkins,' she trilled, quickly heading out of his office and towards the school gates.

Mr Hopkins called after her. 'Oh, frabjous day! Miss Drummond, will you marry me?' Hermione turned on her heel, open-mouthed, and made no answer. Mr Hopkins joined her at the gates, taking her hands. 'Or, failing that, shall I accompany you to Totley Garage?' he entreated.

Hermione composed herself. 'Mr Hopkins, I have been thinking that at the end of the month I would very much like to go to Viareggio. Have you ever been?'

'I have not. Is that in Italy?'

'It is indeed. Would you like to accompany me?' she proposed.

'A respectable couple like ourselves could only go if we were man and wife.'

'Very well then, if you insist,' Hermione accepted. 'But we'll have to make plans immediately if we're to get a good long break. Are you busy on the 24th of this month?'

'The 24th?'

'It is a Saturday,' Hermione expanded.

'I do not believe I am engaged that day.'

'Well, consider yourself engaged now. We can go directly from the reception to the airport. I will telephone my travel agent in the morning.'

'And the vicar?' he enquired.

'I will leave the ceremony arrangements up to you,' she yielded.

'Shall we go directly to The Good Intent to celebrate, Hermione?'

'Why not?' she replied. 'This is one of life's lovely moments. I may only be your fiancée for a short time but I intend to enjoy it.'

Everyone at the clinic was excited at Hermione's news. Everyone that is except for Mrs Jefferies. On hearing about our colleague's upcoming nuptials, Mrs Jefferies screwed up her face like she was eating a lemon. She slurped her tea thoughtfully before offering her considered opinion on the matter.

'I wouldn't want to be getting used to a man's funny little ways at your age, Miss Drummond. I do think you're brave to take him on and with his health problems,' remarked Mrs Jefferies. 'I suppose there is something to be said for companionship in later years,' she mused begrudgingly.

'Who gives two figs about companionship?' replied Hermione. 'I'm planning on having lots of sex.'

Mrs Jefferies spluttered into her tea and started to cough. 'Well I never …' she started to protest.

'I'm sure you never,' mocked Hermione.

Mrs Jefferies stormed out of the room. Hermione opened her mouth but before she could get her words out, Mrs King, Laura, Nurse Higgins and I all said in unison, 'Saucer of cream for Miss Drummond,' and how we laughed.

# 28

All of the cars were filthy. There wasn't enough water to wash them. Once the summer holidays started most of my home visits were in the back gardens. The mums and I would chat while older children splashed in paddling pools filled up with the left-over washing-up water. The summer drought had scorched the fields and dried up the river beds. Half my mums were not at home at all but in the fields and orchards picking and the usually lively baby clinic became a bit thin on the ground. It seemed like the whole village was picking, even those who didn't need the money.

'What are going to do about it, Hill?' Hermione asked, looking at me over her spectacles perched on the end of her nose while she wrote out the invitations for her wedding.

'If the mountain won't come to Mohammed,' I replied.

'Excellent, quite excellent,' she said with a smile, then licked an envelope written in her beautiful swirly handwriting.

After my morning calls I would drive out to the fields and orchards and visit there. My nifty little scales enabled me to run outdoor baby clinics for the mums while they picked. At Mill Farm it seemed like every tree had a pram parked underneath it for shade, but there were a lot of sunburnt grumpy children about. I raided the clothing boxes to find sun hats and loose T-shirts, and loaded up my Mini with sunscreen and bottles of water in an attempt to keep the mothers and children safe and hydrated. Wherever I rolled up my first job was always to give everyone a big drink before we got down to any feeding, sleep, weaning or behavioural issues. Sid Holleman, kind soul that he was, let me use the weighing tent to see the mothers so we could chat in the cool of the white marquee. I don't think he ever let me leave without a box of fruit.

Hermione's wedding day was a scorcher from first light but heat or no heat, the whole village would turn out to wish Mr Hopkins and Miss Drummond the best of luck. Mrs King and I went down to River Cottage after breakfast to see if Hermione needed any help getting ready. My dear friend had asked me to drive her to the church in her own MG. I had a long shiny blue ribbon in my pocket and Mrs King had brought a beautiful arrangement of deep-pink, hundred-leaved roses for the bride's bouquet and to decorate the car. Trev had let me have the spare set he kept for Hermione and like a pair of mischievous schoolgirls Mrs King and I crept down the driveway where the MG was parked under an open porch, put the top down and decorated the car in a murmur of hushed giggles.

Hermione stood before the mirror of her dressing room. She looked divine in a long dove-grey gown, her hair pulled back softly off her face in waves with diamante hair slides. She had three strings of pearls around her neck that she constantly twiddled with, making knots and then untying them again. She looked like Claudette Colbert in *It Happened One Night*, so tall and elegant, with large dark eyes. Mrs King handed Hermione her bouquet. She dipped her head down into the flora and smelled the roses appreciatively.

'What a gorgeous clear and sweet smell with honey tones. How clever of you to pick these roses, Beatie – you know they mean sincere love,' praised Hermione. 'I didn't imagine I'd ever be a bride. Do I look ridiculous?' she asked, staring at her reflection in the long freestanding oval mirror in a rare moment of self-doubt.

'You look like a queen,' Mrs King told her. 'And a queen of England,' she added.

'In that case, ladies, get me to the church on time,' instructed Hermione.

She was thrilled to see her MG decorated and off we went on the short drive to St Agatha's up Totley Hill. Less than an hour later, Hermione and Mr Hopkins were married.

'I don't think I'll ever be able to call her Mrs Hopkins,' Clem whispered to me in the churchyard as we assembled for the photographs. 'Do you think she could keep on using Miss Drummond professionally, like an actress?'

We followed the happy couple down Main Street and into the Village Hall. Mrs King and Flo had put up bunting and created splendid flower arrangements. Ted from The Good Intent closed the pub for the day to do the catering and bar, a free bar thanks to the generous Mr Hopkins. When we arrived at the hall Ted ran out to Hermione, sweating and very red in the face.

'I'm so sorry, Miss Drummond, er, Mrs Hopkins. The water pipes have swelled in the heat and I can't get any fresh water out, it just comes out brown.'

'No fresh water?' Hermione asked.

'I'm afraid not,' the fretful landlord confirmed.

'Oh well, if we must drink champagne, we must,' said Hermione, laughing with a dramatic shrug.

Mrs King and I were sitting enjoying the coconut wedding cake and coffee when Hermione bustled over.

'Did I tell you I've got two hearing tests booked on Monday? The Wraight baby needs to get a referral from the GP to check his hips. Mrs Lauter on The Meadows estate is having a very hard time with that fella of hers – please do keep an eye on her. Mrs Mires's twins' nursery places need chasing up and there was something else ...' she finished, biting her lip and trying to recall, while drumming her fingers on the wedding table. Her gold wedding ring glistened on her formerly bare finger.

'We know, Hermione. You've left us extensive notes,' Mrs King told her. 'Miss Hill and I are perfectly capable of covering your caseload for a month. Enjoy your honeymoon.'

'Did I tell you about my elderly lady on Fairy Hill?' interrupted Hermione.

'You did,' I said. 'Now I think someone is waiting for you to leave for the airport.'

Hermione glanced over her shoulder. Mr Hopkins was waiting at the door with his hand extended to her. A little crowd assembled to wave them off.

'I'm coming,' Hermione called. 'Line up, ladies, and I'll throw my bouquet.'

Danny watched me closely as I lined up with the other girls. He was heading to Scotland again tomorrow morning. I felt each time he went he left a little bit more of his heart in Glasgow. It was only natural.

As Hermione breezed past she whispered in my ear, 'Go left!'. The bride stood with her back to us and tossed her bouquet of pink roses high into the air. They were coming towards me fast. I reached up my hands to catch them but Laura Bates's nimble hands shot in front of my face and snatched them away. The district nurse jumped up and down, giddy with anticipation. 'Two more moons, just two more moons,' she told me. I thought back to the rosebush Queenie Dangerfield had given her. Rather you than me, Laura, and I wished her luck.

My romances always seemed to fizzle out.

# 29

There were only two more days to go till the village fete. I waited for Mr and Mrs Reyes to come to the side gate at Totley Grange on Thursday afternoon but it was gone five o'clock and still no sign of them. The previous week their airline tickets had arrived just in time. It was now or never: if we didn't take our chance on Saturday they would have to apply again for a visa which they couldn't afford and Mrs Reyes's sister was unlikely to pay for more airline tickets. Could I go up to the house on some pretext, I wondered. I turned my Mini around and drove up to the big house. Unfortunately, the door was opened by Lady Cecilia herself.

'Miss Hill. You've called at a rather inconvenient time. Did you need to speak to me about your duties for the fete on Saturday?' she asked, barring the threshold.

'Yes,' I breezed. 'I went to Treetops Farm this morning. They're making the hay bales and I asked Mrs Rudcliff whether they could spare a few for the fete.' Mandy Rudcliff had offered them for the Mothers' Interest Group to put on a little café but up until that moment I'd had no intention of asking for her ladyship's permission.

'In what way would bales of hay be useful?' enquired Lady Cecilia sniffily.

'Some of the mums thought it would make a nice rustic café for the children. Keep them out of the tea tent by offering little cakes and bottles of pop.'

Lady Cecilia contemplated my suggestion. 'The children are rather a nuisance in the tea tent. I seem to recall one of that mechanic's children knocking over my Pimm's cup last year. Yes, why not. Is there anything else?' she asked, half closing the door.

'No, no. I just wanted your opinion before I asked Mr Rudcliff to deliver the hay. Would nine o'clock on Saturday morning work?'

'Yes. Tell him to set them on the village green by The Good Intent. It's the more raucous end of things.'

'Certainly, Lady Cecilia. Thank you for your time. While I'm here I haven't seen the Reyeses' baby for a few months and I do need to keep an eye on my caseload.'

Lady Cecilia sighed. 'You'd better come in then. But you can only have 10 minutes. I've got so much to do, I can't have Cristina neglecting her duties.'

I followed Lady Cecilia to the garden. Mr and Mrs Reyes were erecting a huge marquee on the lawn at the back of the house that sloped down to the river. 'We're planning a little party on Saturday night. I sent the veterinary an invitation but I've not had a reply. Has he mentioned it?' He'd mentioned it all right – rubbing elbows with the county set had certainly lost its appeal for Danny. I was surprised though that he hadn't sent his apologies.

'Regretfully he's on call Saturday night,' I lied. I didn't know if he was or not, I wasn't his social secretary. I glowered on the inside.

'How disappointing. We're putting Dash to stud and we hoped he would talk him up to some interested parties,' Lady Cecilia complained.

'He'll be so sorry to miss that. I'll just pop over and see the baby.' Where was Crystal, I suddenly wondered. Mrs Reyes had taken to carrying her baby about in a wrap while she did her work to keep her daughter close but she couldn't do that while erecting a huge flipping tent and I didn't spy Crystal's basket anywhere.

'Cristina has finally seen sense. I insisted she leave the baby under a tree in the orchard. She cried a bit but she'll soon learn not to,' Lady Cecilia informed me. Did she mean baby Crystal or her mother? Probably both, I concluded. 'Chop, chop, Cristina. You've 200 scones to bake before you make dinner.' She turned to me with a benevolent smile. 'I'm donating them for the tea tent,' she explained.

'How generous,' I replied through a forced smile.

I trotted over to the Reyeses. Mrs Reyes led me to the orchard while her husband remained under the watchful eye of his employers struggling with tent poles. We followed Crystal's cries to underneath a cherry tree. Mrs Reyes reached in and hugged her baby tight.

'Not long, my baby, not long now,' Cristina Reyes whispered, kissing the top of her child's soft dark head.

'We don't have much time, I'm afraid. Have you got everything packed and ready for Saturday?' I asked.

'Yes. We aren't allowed to go to the fete on Saturday. It's not our day off and we have to get everything ready for the party.'

'Both Lady Cecilia and the Captain will be there to open the fete on Saturday afternoon, won't they?'

'Yes. We don't expect them back till six o'clock.'

'Will there be anybody else in the house?'

'Master Bertie is about. I doubt he'll show his face in the village at the moment. But he often drives to London to a party on the weekend but he doesn't get up till lunchtime.'

'I'll come and pick you up at two o'clock. That'll give me time to taste all the jams and be back at three o'clock to give out the prize.'

'What if something goes wrong?'

'We just have to keep our heads and hope it won't. You're almost there, Cristina. Only two more nights and you'll be on your way to America.'

The straw bales were practically the same colour as the grass on the village green. We'd not had a drop of rain for weeks and the hot weather had become too close for comfort. The air felt electric with heat and energy and so did I. I licked my lips thoughtfully, tasting each jam carefully and making notes on a score sheet while Hermione, fresh from a steamy honeymoon in Viareggio, inspected the sweet peas and Mrs King's discerning palate sampled the scones.

Every member of the Totley WI had gathered outside the tent while we remained locked inside behind secured flaps until it was all finished. There wasn't enough air in the tent and I was keen to be off. After selecting first, second and third place I slipped out as Mrs Jefferies was judging the beautiful baby competition. Fisticuffs had already broken out when she informed Carol Mires that her Alan had a squint. He most certainly did not. My critical colleague had picked the wrong mother to mess with, as I knew from first-hand experience.

I parked my Mini at the side of Totley Grange. It was almost two o'clock. The kitchen door opened and Mr Reyes crept out with a single suitcase holding Crystal, who was sleepy and getting cross in the heat. He opened the door very quietly and got into the back seat with the baby.

'Anything else?' I asked.

'No, just my wife,' he replied, his face furrowed with worry.

'Where is she?'

'We were just about to leave when Master Bertie came into the kitchen demanding breakfast. He's still drunk from last night. She's cooking him eggs and bacon now,' José Reyes explained.

'He can't stop her,' I said. 'It doesn't matter if they sack you now, you don't need their job,' I said boldly.

'No, but you do. If Lady Cecilia and the Captain find out you've been helping us I imagine she would make life very difficult for you.'

It was true she would.

'That doesn't matter. I don't want you to miss your train.' I looked anxiously at the clock.

'Let's wait a few more minutes,' he pressed.

The time seemed to go far too slowly. I worried something had happened. It was almost 2.15 p.m. We wound all the windows down and tried to fan Crystal with a newspaper as she grew ever more fractious in the afternoon sun. I needed to get them onto the train at 2.30 p.m. and get back to the fete without anyone noticing I'd gone. The kitchen door opened and to my everlasting relief Cristina emerged. She was dressed in a simple floral summer frock Hermione had given her – I'd never seen her look so lovely. She carried her black maid's uniform in her arms and as she passed the dustbin lifted the lid and threw it in. Mr Reyes and I gave a low cheer.

'He's gone back to bed. Quick, let's go before he wants something else,' she said.

I didn't need telling twice. We sped off to Totley Station just in time for the London train. I walked with them to the platform and watched as they got into the second-class carriage and waved them off to London Heathrow and a fairer life, I hoped. If I'd only done one good thing during my first year as a health visitor I was certain it was this.

*　*　*

I parked my trusty green Mini at Ivy Cottage and walked very quickly back to the fete, feeling rather sticky but completely exhilarated. Danny saw me, winked and ran over to meet me.

'Been playing hooky, have we?' he asked, jogging next to me as I pressed on to the stage.

'I just popped home to use the loo,' I said.

'I've been looking for you for over an hour. Lady Cecilia is insisting we go to that flaming party. I don't know if I can afford to snub her,' Danny said, frowning.

'We can go if you like but I think it will be a bit of a flop.'

'Why?'

'Just a feeling.'

'A fortune teller, are you? Some of that gypsy magic must have rubbed off.'

'They should have had Queenie Dangerfield to tell fortunes.'

'The WI would never allow it.'

'Oh really. I've passed many a respectable lady coming out of Queenie's caravan when they were at Mill Farm.'

'*Do* tell!'

'I couldn't possibly. Shush! They're going to announce the judging.' I elbowed him in the ribs.

Lady Cecilia announced each prize winner into the microphone as we stood huddled together in the oppressive heat, fanning ourselves with hats and fans, desperate for her to finish so we could go to the pub. As she dismounted the stage her son screeched up onto the green, leaving tyre marks in the frazzled lawn to much tut-tutting.

'Mother,' he called. 'Those Filipinos have hopped it.' He frantically waved a note in the air.

'Hush, Bertie, what are you talking about?' snapped Lady Cecilia, trying to quieten him down but for once the crowd were all ears.

'I came down to get another helping of bacon and eggs and some coffee and the woman wasn't there. I saw this note on the kitchen table, so I opened it, and look,' he informed her ladyship, passing her the letter.

As she read the note, Lady Cecilia's face turned crimson from her throat to the tips of her ears. 'They've gone to work for someone else with no forwarding address. After all we've done for them,' she railed. 'Of all the nerve. You just can't trust a certain sort of people,' she said, tearing up the letter into little pieces. 'Did they leave everything ready for the party?' Her son shook his head.

I had to look in the other direction so Lady Cecilia wouldn't see me smile. A huge bolt of lightning tore across the sky followed by a clap of thunder and the whole of Totley held their breath in one moment of anticipation. The heavens opened and the cool summer rain fell onto the crowd. No one ran for cover; we opened our arms and let the rain wash over us. The band broke into a chorus of 'Here Comes the Sun' and we danced in the rain until we were wet through.

It had been a year since I came to Totley and I'd learnt so much from all those babies and their wonderful mothers. I couldn't wait to see what my second year as a health visitor would bring.

# Acknowledgements

Thanks to fellow health visitors and friends in Kent and Staffordshire over the decades, especially Daphne Claw, Catherine Powell, Alana Macgregor and Lynne Keane. Knocking on people's doors is never easy, and your humour, warmth and camaraderie through the years is what makes nurses such good friends. Not forgetting Carmel and Hugh Glennie and Peggy Johnson for being there from the very beginning.

To Margaret Jehu, Paul Magrs and Mark Beyer-Kay for your wonderful insights into writing and life. People who are not only talented themselves but unlock the potential in others truly make the world a better place.

To Divya Venkatesh for helping to give illustrative form to our ideas, Dr Emma Nicholas for veterinary advice and Nikki Dore for sharing mystical secrets.

Thank you to the staff at the National Archives, Museum for English Rural Life, Kent History & Library Centre, BBC Archives and the Royal Institution of Great Britain for keeping such meticulous records.

To all the readers of *The New Arrival* who got in touch to let us know how much you enjoyed the first book: your encouragement and support makes such a difference, and readers are always welcome to connect with us at sarahbeeson.org.

To Takbir Uddin for always being able to make us laugh, and Ava who started this journey and is the reason for everything.

*Sarah and Amy Beeson*

# Also by Sarah Beeson

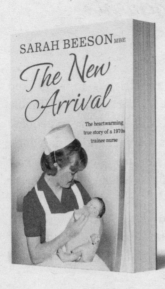

Sarah Beeson's poignant memoir captures both the heartache and happiness of hospital life and 1970s London through the eyes of a gentle but determined young nurse.

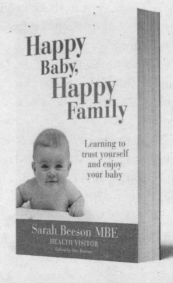

With Sarah Beeson's book to hand you have a best friend with great advice and a gentle approach to guide you through your baby's first year.